Revisional Surgery

Editor

SEAN T. GRAMBART

CLINICS IN PODIATRIC MEDICINE AND SURGERY

www.podiatric.theclinics.com

Consulting Editor
THOMAS J. CHANG

July 2020 • Volume 37 • Number 3

ELSEVIER

1600 John F. Kennedy Boulevard • Suite 1800 • Philadelphia, Pennsylvania, 19103-2899

http://www.theclinics.com

CLINICS IN PODIATRIC MEDICINE AND SURGERY Volume 37, Number 3
July 2020 ISSN 0891-8422, ISBN-13: 978-0-323-77626-4

Editor: Lauren Boyle
Developmental Editor: Nicole Congleton

Clinics in Podiatric Medicine and Surgery (ISSN 0891-8422) is published quarterly by Elsevier Inc., 360 Park Avenue South, New York, NY 10010-1710. Months of issue are January, April, July, and October. Business and Editorial Offices: 1600 John F. Kennedy Blvd., Ste. 1800, Philadelphia, PA 19103-2899. Customer Service Office: 3251 Riverport Lane, Maryland Heights, MO 63043. Periodicals postage paid at New York, NY and additional mailing offices. Subscription prices are $304.00 per year for US individuals, $597.00 per year for US institutions, $100.00 per year for US students and residents, $382.00 per year for Canadian individuals, $721.00 for Canadian institutions, $457.00 for international individuals, $721.00 per year for international institutions, $100.00 per year for Canadian students/residents, and $220.00 per year for foreign students/residents. To receive student/resident rate, orders must be accompanied by name of affiliated institution, date of term, and the *signature* of program/residency coordinator on institution letterhead. Orders will be billed at individual rate until proof of status is received. Foreign air speed delivery is included in all *Clinics* subscription prices. All prices are subject to change without notice. POSTMASTER: Send address changes to *Clinics in Podiatric Medicine and Surgery*, Elsevier Health Sciences Division, Subscription Customer Service, 3251 Riverport Lane, Maryland Heights, MO 63043. **Customer Service: 1-800-654-2452 (US). From outside of the US, call 314-447-8871. Fax: 314-447-8029. E-mail: JournalsCustomerService-usa@elsevier.com (for print support); JournalsOnlineSupport-usa@elsevier.com (for online support).**

Reprints. For copies of 100 or more of articles in this publication, please contact the Commercial Reprints Department, Elsevier Inc., 360 Park Avenue South, New York, NY 10010-1710. Tel.: 212-633-3874; Fax: 212-633-3820; E-mail: reprints@elsevier.com.

Clinics in Podiatric Medicine and Surgery is covered in *MEDLINE/PubMed (Index Medicus)* and *EMBASE/Excerpta Medica*.

Contributors

CONSULTING EDITOR

THOMAS J. CHANG, DPM
Clinical Professor and Past Chairman, Department of Podiatric Surgery, California College of Podiatric Medicine, Faculty, The Podiatry Institute, Redwood Orthopedic Surgery Associates, Santa Rosa, California

EDITOR

SEAN T. GRAMBART, DPM, FACFAS
Assistant Professor, Des Moines University, College of Podiatric Medicine and Surgery, Attending Physician, Unitypoint Health - Iowa Methodist Medical Center, Des Moines, Iowa

AUTHORS

TRAVIS DREW ANDERSON, BS
Podiatric Medical Student, Des Moines University, College of Podiatric Medicine and Surgery, Des Moines, Iowa

DANIKA S. ANDERSON, BS
Podiatric Medical Student, Des Moines University, College of Podiatric Medicine and Surgery, Des Moines, Iowa

ERIC A. BARP, DPM, FACFAS
Attending Physician, The Iowa Clinic, Unitypoint Health, Des Moines, Iowa

MARY BRANDT, BA
Podiatric Medical Student, Des Moines University, Des Moines, Iowa

JOSEPH R. BROWN, BS
Podiatric Medical Student, Des Moines University, College of Podiatric Medicine and Surgery, Des Moines, Iowa

DONALD E. BUDDECKE, Jr, DPM, FACFAS
Private Practice, Foot & Ankle Specialists, PC, Omaha, Nebraska

KATHERINE FRUSH, DPM, FACFAS
Associate Professor, Des Moines University, College of Podiatric Medicine and Surgery, Des Moines, Iowa

SEAN T. GRAMBART, DPM, FACFAS
Assistant Professor, Des Moines University, College of Podiatric Medicine and Surgery, Attending Physician, Unitypoint Health - Iowa Methodist Medical Center, Des Moines, Iowa

BYRON HUTCHINSON, DPM, FACFAS
Director, Advanced Foot & Ankle Fellowship, CHI Franciscan, Burien, Washington

NEPHI E.H. JONES, DPM, PGY2
Resident Physician, Unitypoint Health - Iowa Methodist Medical Center, Des Moines, Iowa

ERIN NELSON, DPM, FACFAS
Assistant Professor and Clinical Chair, Des Moines University, Des Moines, Iowa

SCOTT C. NELSON, DPM, FACFAS
Department of Orthopedics, Catholic Health Initiatives (CHI Health), Omaha, Nebraska

GARRETT B. NGUYEN, DPM
Resident Physician, Department of Podiatric Surgery, AdventHealth East Orlando Podiatric Surgery Residency, Orlando, Florida

AMANDA NIESTER, BS, DPM
21 Student, Des Moines University, College of Podiatric Medicine and Surgery, Des Moines, Iowa

RYAN D. PRUSA, DPM, PGY1
Resident Physician, Unitypoint Health - Iowa Methodist Medical Center, Des Moines, Iowa

ERIC R. REESE, DPM
Chief Resident, Unitypoint Health - Iowa Methodist Medical Center, Des Moines, Iowa

CHRISTOPHER L. REEVES, DPM, FACFAS
Faculty and Director of Research, Podiatric Surgery Residency, AdventHealth East Orlando, Orlando Foot and Ankle Clinic–Upperline Health, Winter Park, Florida

THOMAS S. ROUKIS, DPM, PhD, FACFAS
Attending Staff, Orthopaedic Center, Gundersen Health System, La Crosse, Wisconsin

HANNAH SAHLI, DPM
Chief Resident, Department of Podiatric Surgery, AdventHealth System, Orlando, Florida

MALLORY J. SCHWEITZER, DPM, MHA
Fellow, Advanced Foot & Ankle Fellowship, CHI Franciscan, Burien, Washington

JOSHUA A. SEBAG, DPM
Chief Resident Physician, Department of Podiatric Surgery, AdventHealth East Orlando Podiatric Surgery Residency, Florida

AMBER M. SHANE, DPM, FACFAS
Chair, Department of Podiatric Surgery, AdventHealth System, Faculty, AdventHealth East Orlando Podiatric Surgery Residency, Orlando Foot and Ankle Clinic - Upperline Health, Orlando, Florida

KATHERINE M. TERNENT, BA
Podiatric Medical Student, Des Moines University, College of Podiatric Medicine and Surgery, Des Moines, Iowa

MITCHELL J. THOMPSON, DPM
PGY-3, Podiatric Medicine and Surgery Resident, Gundersen Medical Foundation, Gundersen Health System, La Crosse, Wisconsin

CODY TOGHER, DPM
Resident, Department of Podiatric Surgery, AdventHealth System, Orlando, Florida

Contents

> Revision surgeries, as well as conversions from implants to arthrodesis, can present unique challenges to the foot and ankle surgeon. Proper perioperative planning assists in optimizing the outcome of the procedure. In general, some amount of bone loss and/or shortening of the first metatarsal takes place, leading to the need for augmenting the site with bone graft or a synthetic substitute. Fixation also plays a key role in obtaining a successful conversion. A solid construct combined with bone graft assists the foot and ankle surgeon in achieving an optimal outcome.

> Revision hammertoe surgery can be extremely challenging for the foot and ankle surgeon given the scar tissue and available osseous and soft tissue. Although not a common procedure, lesser metatarsophalangeal joint arthrodesis is an option for the patient especially in lieu of an amputation. This article describes the current literature and the surgical technique for a lesser metatarsophalangeal joint arthrodesis.

> Nonunion of the tarsometatarsal arthrodesis site is a challenging revision surgery. Trephine technique provides an excellent option for revision tarsometatarsal joint arthrodesis. The authors have found the trephine approach to be the procedure of choice in correction of a nonunion. When the trephine approach is indicated, it offers many advantages including minimal soft tissue dissection, quicker joint preparation, and the minimal shortening of the arthrodesis site. This article describes in detail the autologous graft trephine technique for revision surgery of a tarsometatarsal nonunion. Examples of fixation options are also discussed.

> Although most primary lateral ankle ligament repairs have a high success rate, as with any surgery, failures and the need for revision can occur.

Nonanatomic lateral ankle ligament repairs have fallen out of favor because of the increased stiffness and resultant change in mechanics of the functioning tendon that is normally used. Allograft anatomic lateral ankle ligament reconstruction for revision surgery has gained popularity over the last few years. This article discusses the factors that can lead to failure and the revision technique.

A malaligned ankle arthrodesis is a painful and complicated pathology. Deformities may be present in the frontal, sagittal, or transverse plane or a combination of planes. Thorough preoperative evaluation of the deformity and the patient as a whole is crucial to successful revision. Surgical site for revision should be based on center of rotation of angulation, when possible. Revision commonly is performed through opening wedge osteotomy. Closing wedge and focal dome osteotomies, however, are excellent options. Revision also may be performed through external fixation or total ankle replacement. Although the literature is not rich with data, the options discussed provide favorable results.

Revision surgery for failed total ankle replacement is a challenge to the revision surgeon. Deformity, presence of infection, segmental bone defects, patient comorbidities, and soft tissue compromise all are significant considerations when determining appropriate procedures. Revision total ankle replacement, explant and fusion with or without lengthening, use of a trabecular metal cage, placement of an antibiotic cement spacer, grafting, and amputation all are viable options to treat patients with failed ankle arthroplasty.

Lapidus arthrodesis is becoming more of a common procedure for treatment of hallux valgus deformities. Like other procedures, complications are possible. The common complications associated with Lapidus arthrodesis procedures include nonunion and malunion. Malunion is typically broken down into recurrence, elevated first ray, shortened first ray, or plantarflexed first ray. This article discusses these common complications after Lapidus arthrodesis.

Forefoot neuromas are a common pathology that is seen in a wide variety of patients. Although conservative treatment is successful with modification of shoes/inserts or injections, surgical intervention is occasionally needed to alleviate the discomfort. Most surgical procedures for neuromas have a good outcome. There are times when the outcome is not optimal and revision surgery may be needed. This article describes revision surgery techniques that may lead to an improved outcome. Also discussed is the opportunity to reduce recurrence through the understanding of neuroma biology, diagnosis, and treatment options.

Osteochondral lesion of the talar dome (OCLT) can be a devastating injury that affects mobility. Etiology of these lesions is debated but trauma seems the most supported etiology. Diagnosis of lesions is based on imaging. Conservative management, including weight-bearing restrictions, physical therapy, and supportive measures, often is first-line treatment. Nonsurgical modalities have mixed results and surgical measures often are necessitated for symptom relief. Surgical treatments vary in invasiveness and often are dictated by OCLT size. Studies show patient satisfaction increases substantially after having these procedures performed after failing nonsurgical measures. Results are encouraging, although thorough workup and discussion should be undertaken.

Treatment of Achilles tendon ruptures may be surgical or nonsurgical depending on health, history, age, acuity, and severity of the injury. With chronic or revisional injuries, the best method often requires an open repair with reconstructive soft tissue procedures. Revision surgery can be challenging because of the complexity involving tendinous deficits with nonviable and friable tissue. Surgical treatment is based on tendon approximation, size of the defect, tendon integrity, and functional demands. The goal is to restore anatomic and physiologic tension, provide adequate strength for proper ambulation, optimize functional return to activity, decrease pain, and decrease complications.

Peroneal tendon tears that require revision are rare and often present a unique challenge for foot and ankle surgeons. Biomechanical issues that may be present or missed initially need to be addressed and evaluated thoroughly for an optimized outcome. Tendon degeneration is usually present, and planning for tendon transfer or tendon graft is necessary to improve mechanical strength. The use of MRI can aid in preoperative planning and identification of concomitant disorders that may be present. The postoperative rehabilitation is often longer and patient education is imperative to manage expectations of outcomes.

Optimal healing for fractures requires anatomic reduction and stable fixation. This optimizes not only bone healing, but optimal function within the

CLINICS IN PODIATRIC MEDICINE AND SURGERY

FORTHCOMING ISSUES

October 2020
Orthoplastic Techniques for Lower Extremity Reconstruction
Edgardo R. Rodriguez-Collazo
and Suhail Masadeh, *Editors*

January 2021
Posterior and Plantar Heel Pain
Eric A. Barp, *Editor*

RECENT ISSUES

April 2020
Innovative Research in Podiatric Medical Schools
Thomas J. Chang, *Editor*

January 2020
Biomechanics of the Lower Extremity
Jarrod Shapiro, *Editor*

SERIES OF RELATED INTEREST

Foot and Ankle Clinics
Orthopedic Clinics

Foreword

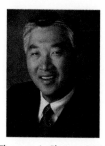

Thomas J. Chang, DPM
Consulting Editor

I am excited to present this current issue on principles and concepts of *Revisional Surgery*. Many of the surgical principles we learn and follow for primary surgery are repeatedly reinforced throughout our training, well practiced throughout our surgical careers, and well ingrained by repetition as they become second nature in time. These can change significantly when dealing with a revision surgery, as soft tissue integrity, neurovascular support, and bone health are often altered. The revisional cases require more preparation and will bring additional stress into our busy lives. These are all challenging and where true education takes place. Some will say "Game On," yet we need to proceed with caution and confidence, and most importantly, take the time to *Be Prepared*. We prepare more rigorously, consulting literature and discussing these cases with multiple colleagues. We will visualize each step of the case and replay this over and over again, so we are able to anticipate any potential surprises. We will also be ready with additional surgical products: orthobiologics, hardware, devices, and stronger fixation constructs.

When these cases are tackled, each opportunity provides tremendous surgical exposure and growth. These cases are where we will learn the most and mature the quickest in our surgical experiences. Even for the experienced surgeon, each opportunity will continue to educate and fine-tune our skills.

I am grateful to Dr Grambart for his guidance and commitment in providing us a variety of challenging topics and talented authors. It is my hope this issue will become a part of your preparation as you consider successful solutions to these difficult cases. Best of luck.

Thomas J. Chang, DPM
Redwood Orthopedic Surgery Associates
208 Concourse Boulevard
Santa Rosa, CA 95403, USA

E-mail address:
thomaschang14@comcast.net

Preface

Not Everything in Life (or Surgery) Is a Guarantee

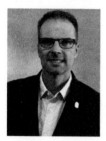

Sean T. Grambart, DPM, FACFAS
Editor

It has been a pleasure to be the guest editor for this issue of *Clinics in Podiatric Medicine and Surgery*. I would first like to thank the authors for their time and expertise. Their desire to educate, share their experiences, and publish continues to help drive our profession forward.

The vast majority of the foot and ankle surgeries that are performed has a high success rate and good to excellent surgical outcomes for our patients. Unfortunately, with any surgical procedure, unexpected and poor surgical outcomes can occur. With these less than desirable outcomes, revision surgery may be necessary. Revision surgery has always been a challenge due to a variety of factors, such as poor bone and soft tissue quality as well as patient expectations. Despite these factors, it is also an excellent educational opportunity for surgeons of all levels.

As I look back on my residency, I was fortunate have many talented surgeons stress the importance of surgical technique. The procedures that were performed on patients that had not had previous surgery aided me in developing my surgical skills. However, what taught me the most about surgery and how to be a surgeon were the cases that challenged me and my attendings to think "outside of the box". More likely than not, these cases were the revision surgery cases.

The hope of this issue on Revisional Surgery is to be an aid to help with these complex procedures. I would like to dedicate this issue to the future surgeons of our

Clin Podiatr Med Surg 37 (2020) xv–xvi
https://doi.org/10.1016/j.cpm.2020.04.001
0891-8422/20/© 2020 Published by Elsevier Inc.

profession. As you go through your educational training, play close attention to the cases that do not go as expected...that is when you will learn the most.

Sean T. Grambart, DPM, FACFAS
College of Podiatric Medicine and Surgery
Des Moines University
3200 Grand Avenue
Des Moines, IA 50312, USA

Unitypoint Health
Iowa Methodist Medical Center
1200 Pleasant Street
Des Moines, IA 50309, USA

E-mail address:
Sean.Grambart@dmu.edu

Revision of Failed First Metatarsophalangeal Joint Implant

Eric A. Barp, DPM[a],*, Nephi E.H. Jones, DPM, PGY2[b],
Ryan D. Prusa, DPM, PGY1[b]

KEYWORDS

- First metatarsophalangeal joint • Arthrodesis • Revision surgery • Failed implants

KEY POINTS

- Autogenous, allogenic, or synthetic bone graft should be incorporated into the surgical plan for implant conversion to arthrodesis of the first metatarsophalangeal joint.
- The optimal fixation for arthrodesis should include a construct that biomechanically provides strength and stability to minimize pain with ambulation after union.
- Maintain open communication between the foot and ankle surgeon and the patient about procedure expectations, realistic goals, and the potential for multiple surgeries.

INTRODUCTION

Surgical options for end-stage hallux rigidus include resection arthroplasty, joint replacement (implants), and arthrodesis.[1] A study by Stone and colleagues[2] in 2017 looked at long-term results of patients randomly assigned to either arthrodesis or total joint arthroplasty groups for hallux rigidus. The results showed lower pain scale ratings, higher satisfaction scores, and fewer revisions in the arthrodesis group. Of the 36 patients in the arthroplasty group, 6 went on to revision arthrodesis, whereas only 1 of the 30 arthrodesis cases required revision. Despite these rates of revision, first metatarsophalangeal joint (MTPJ) arthroplasties have gained high popularity among foot and ankle surgeons over the years, with an increasing number of implantable materials and constructs for treatment of hallux rigidus. Results of implant arthroplasties have been largely inconsistent with some unacceptably high failure rates mixed with some reported excellent outcomes.[3,4] Patients with excellent results need to understand that implant arthroplasty may not last a lifetime and revision is a

[a] The Iowa Clinic, Unitypoint Health, 5950 University Avenue West, Des Moines, IA 50266, USA;
[b] Unitypoint Health - Iowa Methodist Medical Center, 1200 Pleasant Street, Des Moines, IA 50309, USA
* Corresponding author.
E-mail address: ebarp@iowaclinic.com

Clin Podiatr Med Surg 37 (2020) 421–431
https://doi.org/10.1016/j.cpm.2020.03.009
0891-8422/20/© 2020 Elsevier Inc. All rights reserved.

possibility at some point. Some implants will fail sooner than expected and require attempted revision or removal with conversion to a first MTPJ arthrodesis. The foot and ankle surgeon must have a proper surgical plan when a revision surgery is needed.

The MTPJ implant constructs take many forms to include hemi-implants (1 side of the joint), total implants (metatarsal head, proximal phalanx base), or synthetic interpositional arthroplasty.[4] When performing these procedures, there is always some degree of bone loss during the procedure. When these ultimately fail, we are left with a shortened first ray, and sometimes, large deficits/voids to fill.[4]

SURGICAL DECISION MAKING

When evaluating a patient for revision surgery after a failed first MTPJ arthroplasty, it is imperative that the surgeon and patient maintain effective communication about realistic goals, expectations, and the potential for multiple surgeries. There are many variables that make revision surgeries much more complicated than the original case that can include poor bone quality, bone loss, and infection. Infection of the implant needs to ruled out with preoperative laboratory work and possible advanced imaging. In cases of infection, the revision surgery will most likely need to be staged to optimize the chance for a successful outcome. The goal of revision surgery should be to restore a functional, stable, and pain-free foot for ambulation.

The majority of the published literature surrounding options for failed first MTPJ arthroplasties (implants, Keller arthroplasty, etc) have advocated that the most appropriate treatment option is to proceed with a first MTPJ arthrodesis with either autologous or allogeneic bone grafting. It has been advocated that first MTPJ arthrodesis provides the length and alignment necessary to facilitate a more stable and functional foot.[5] Considerations before performing conversion to arthrodesis include the need for bone graft (allograft, autologous, or synthetic) as well as appropriate fixation options. The decision on the bone graft can often be debated. There are options for using autologous versus allogeneic and cortical versus cancellous bone. Even the location for the autologous graft can be a topic of debate.

Autogenic bone grafts are the most preferred; however, depending on the harvested location, not all provide structural support and help to maintain length at the fusion site. The major locations for harvesting bone graft for foot and ankle surgery are the iliac crest, fibula, proximal tibia, and the calcaneus. Autogenic bone grafts provide osteogenic, osteoconductive, and osteoinductive properties that can ultimately provide the optimal healing environment.[6,7] However, there are disadvantages to autogenous bone grafts, including the risks with the secondary harvest procedures to include seromas, hematomas, nerve damage, infection, and fracture.[6–8] Although the harvest risk are not present for allografts, allogenic or synthetic grafts do not provide all the properties that autografts afford.

Structural bone grafts, such as tricortical iliac bone, fibular bone sections, and cadaveric femoral head, provide stability and help to restore the desired length of the first ray.[7,9,10] Cancellous bone grafts (usually harvested from the proximal tibia or calcaneus) as well as synthetic or bone graft substitutes are useful for augmenting the fusion site; however, they provide little stability or structure.[6,7]

Proper preoperative planning through plain radiographs or advanced imaging (computed tomography scans, MRI) along with knowing the type of implant (hemi, total, or synthetic interposition) will allow the surgeon to plan for the appropriate bone graft selection for optimal results.

The type of implant that was used can also give the surgeon direction on the most appropriate fixation options when undertaking the revision arthrodesis. For synthetic interpositional implants, the surgeon can consider a wider range of fixation options (crossing screws, K-wires, or combination screws, staples, and/or plates) because there is often a limited loss of length and bone after removal of these implants. Similarly with hemi-implants on the proximal phalanx base, conventional options could still be considered. For total and metatarsal head implants, the surgeon should recognize the potential for significant bone loss and shortening of the first ray.[11] In these cases, a structural bone graft with plate fixation could be more optimal.

Moon and McGlamry[12] in 2011 presented fixation options for first MTPJ arthrodesis. They extensively reviewed fixation options to include Kirschner wires/Steinmann pin fixation, screw fixation, plate fixation, compression screw with plate, staple fixation, and external fixation. They found equally high rates of union between all types of fixation. Biomechanically, they found that more structurally sound types of fixation (interfragmentary screws with plate) showed increased strength and stability.

It is also important to briefly mention locking plates versus nonlocking plates. There are several advantages of a locking plate system. Locking plates do not require precise bending or adaptation to the underlying bone. Unlike conventional plating systems, locking plates do not draw the bone segments to the plate when tightening the screws, thus decreasing the risk of altering the reduction. Conventional plates compress the cortical bone, which could lead to disruption of perfusion. Locking plate systems are designed to decrease this compressive force and the risk of cortical perfusion embarrassment. Another advantage that locking plates have over conventional plates is the decreased risk of loosening screws, especially when a bone graft

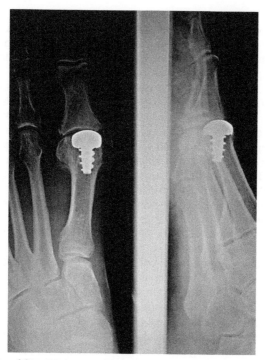

Fig. 1. Radiographs of first MPJ implant failure.

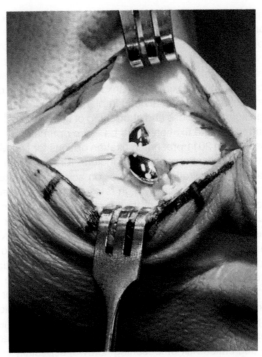

Fig. 2. Failed implant as seen through standard incisional approach to the first MPJ.

is being incorporated. The final advantage of using a locking plate is that they provide a more stable and rigid fixation. Some foot and ankle surgeons might argue that too rigid of a construct will not allow for callus formation and lead to a delayed or nonunion in some situations.

There is limited published research comparing locking versus nonlocking plating systems for first MTPJ arthrodesis. The limited evidence that is available is somewhat conflicting. Hunt and colleagues[13] published a study comparing locking plates versus nonlocking plates of first MTPJ arthrodesis and reported a nonunion rate of 22.8% for locking plate group (16/73) compared with 11.4% for nonlocking group (13/107). In contrast, Doty and colleagues[14] reported a 98% (45/46) fusion rate and Mann and colleagues[15] reported a 95.24% (20/21) fusion rate while using a locking plate with a lag screw for first MTPJ arthrodesis. More investigation should be undertaken in this comparison because there is insufficient evidence to support the superiority of locking plates versus conventional plates when performing first MTPJ arthrodesis.

Primary research into revision of the failed first MPJ implant is limited. The largest case series to date was published by Usuelli and colleges[16] in 2017 where 12 consecutive patients underwent bone block arthrodesis after failure of first MTPJ replacement. Patients underwent arthrodesis using ipsilateral calcaneal bone graft. Of the 12 patients, 3 (25%) went on to nonunion. One of these was symptomatic and required revision, and the other 2 were asymptomatic and required no additional surgery at the conclusion of the study. Average visual analog scale, satisfaction scores, and functional indexed all improved after surgical intervention. The study concluded that revision arthrodesis is a viable surgical option to improve patient function while avoiding first ray shortening; however, they cautioned readers of a high 25% nonunion rate.

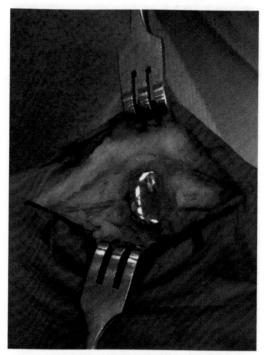

Fig. 3. Implant visualized through dorsomedial incision. Adequate exposure is paramount to achieve optimal alignment, healing, and functional outcomes.

SURGICAL TECHNIQUE

The authors preference for performing first MTPJ arthrodesis following failed first MTPJ implants includes obtaining bone marrow aspirate (BMA) combined with either cancellous bone graft from the calcaneus or femoral head allograft and the use of combined compression (interfragmentary) screw with dorsal locking plate.

Case Report

A 54-year-old woman with a failed arthroplasty of the first MTPJ both clinically and radiographically (**Fig. 1**).

- A Jamshidi needle inserted medial to the tibial tuberosity to harvest approximately 10 mL of BMA from the proximal tibia.
- Exsanguinate the lower extremity and inflate the tourniquet
- Create an approximately 6- to 8-cm incision over the dorsomedial first MTPJ and expose the joint in usual fashion. Adequate exposure is paramount to achieve optimal alignment and functional outcomes (**Figs. 2–4**).
- Remove the implant and all devitalized/nonviable tissue and bone (**Figs. 5 and 6**). There are times when the tourniquet will need to be deflated to determine if the bone is viable or not. Irrigate the joint. Consider sending a sample of bone for pathology to rule out any disease process causing the implant failure.
- Prepare the opposing bone ends for arthrodesis with cup reamers or curettes, irrigate, and then perform subchondral drilling

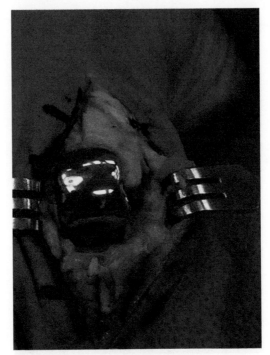

Fig. 4. Implant in situ at the head of the first metatarsal.

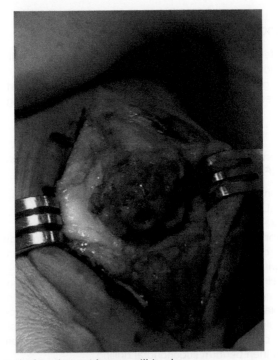

Fig. 5. After removal of implant with stem still in place.

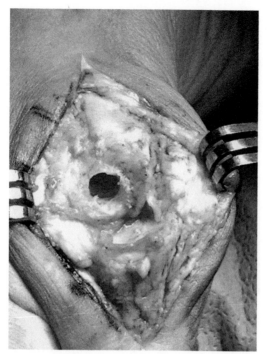

Fig. 6. View of first metatarsal with stem removed. Care must be taken to remove all devitalized/nonviable tissue and bone. A large bone void is present in the metatarsal and proper length has been lost.

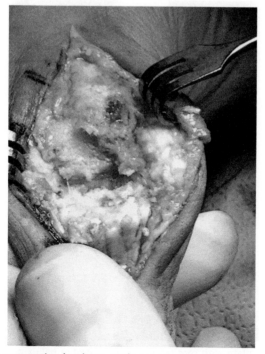

Fig. 7. After bone preparation has been performed.

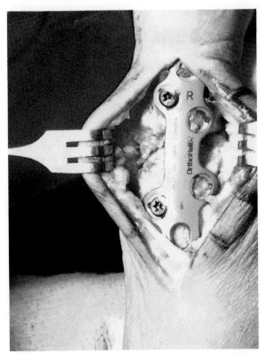

Fig. 8. Placement of plate with care taken to ensure proper hallux position and anatomic length of the first ray.

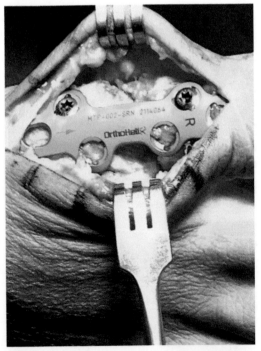

Fig. 9. Placement of plate with care taken to ensure proper hallux position and anatomic length of the first ray.

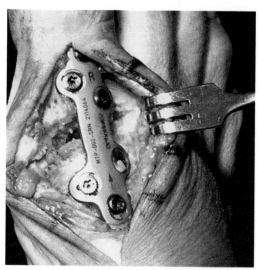

Fig. 10. Medial Oblique View of final plate fixation before graft placement.

- The technique that the authors' use for cancellous graft uses an approximately 1-cm incision over the lateral calcaneus, blunt dissection to the lateral wall of the calcaneus, insert an 8-mm trocar and harvest bone
- When using a structural allograft, the authors recommend the use of a femoral head allograft. Measure the joint space to determine the size of graft needed. Cut the allograft to size.
- In a specimen cup, combine 3 mL of BMA and calcaneus bone graft on the back table (soak the allograft in BMA in a specimen cup).
- Position bone graft into the joint and then position the first MTPJ arthrodesis site so that the hallux if parallel to the second metatarsal, neutral position in the frontal

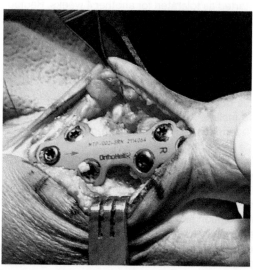

Fig. 11. Lateral Oblique View of final plate fixation before graft placement.

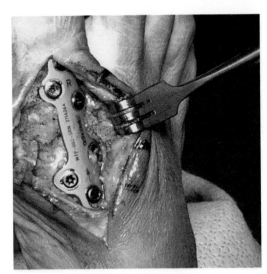

Fig. 12. After graft placement at the arthrodesis site.

plane, and 0° to 10° in the sagittal plane depending on the preference of the surgeon and the patient. Temporarily fix the graft with a K-wire.

- Affix a 6-hole locking plate distally (**Figs. 7–9**). Insert a 4-0 cannulated screw across the joint over the K-wire for compression if there is no need for a structural graft. If a structural graft is needed, then a noncompression screw can be used. Affix the plate proximally. Additional graft can be used as needed to fill any osseous voids (**Figs. 10–12**). Once fixation placement is confirmed on radiographs, layered closure is performed after the area is irrigated.

The postoperative course is nonweightbearing for 4 weeks in a splint or controlled ankle motion boot. If there is radiographic signs of healing, then partial weightbearing in the boot can be started as tolerated for another 4 weeks. Radiographs are repeated at 8 weeks after surgery and the patient can advance out of the boot if everything is stable and healing at that time.

SUMMARY

In recent years, more published literature has emerged discussing the challenges of revision surgeries to include conversion of implant to arthrodesis of the first MTPJ. More investigation needs to be undertaken in regard to fixation because there is still insufficient evidence to support the superiority of 1 fixation option over another when performing first MTPJ arthrodesis. The evidence, however, does support that more advanced types of fixation (an interfragmentary screw with dorsal plating) showed increased strength and stability from a biomechanical standpoint. The foot and ankle surgeon should also perform adequate preoperative planning to include choosing the optimal fixation and choice of bone graft, along with continued communication about realistic expectations and goals with the patient in an attempt to achieve the optimal outcome. The author's preference for conversion of first MTPJ implant to arthrodesis includes BMA, calcaneal bone graft, an interfragmentary compression screw, and a dorsal locking plate.

DISCLOSURE

The authors have nothing to disclose.

REFERENCES

1. Hamilton G, Ford L, Patel S. First metatarsal phalangeal joint arthrodesis and revision arthrodesis. Clin Podiatr Med Surg 2009;26:459–73.
2. Stone O, Ray R, Thomson C, et al. Long-term follow-up of arthrodesis vs total joint arthroplasty for hallux rigidus. Foot Ankle Int 2017;38(4):375–80.
3. Murphay L, Mendicino R, Catanzariti A. Essential insights on first MPJ implant revision. Podiatry Today 2008;21(5).
4. Greisberg J. The Failed First Metatarsophalangeal joint implant arthroplasty. Foot Ankle Clin N Am 2014;19:343–8.
5. Esway J, Conti S. Joint replacement in the hallux metatarsophalangeal joint. Foot Ankle Clin N Am 2005;10:97–115.
6. Mahan K, Hillstrom H. Bone grafting in foot and ankle surgery, a review of 300 cases. J Am Podiatr Med Assoc 1998;88(3):109–18.
7. Roukis T. First metatarsal-phalangeal joint arthrodesis: primary, revision, and salvage of complications. Clin Podiatr Med Surg 2017;34:301–14.
8. Mendicino RW, Leonheart E, Shromoff P. Techniques for harvesting autogenous bone grafts of the lower extremity. J Foot Ankle Surg 1996;35(5):428–35.
9. Lombardi C, Silhanek A, Connolly F, et al. First metatarsophalangeal arthrodesis for treatment of hallux rigidus: a retrospective study. J Foot Ankle Surg 2001; 40(3):137–43.
10. Myerson M, Schon L, McGuigan F, et al. Result of arthrodesis of the hallux metatarsophalangeal joint using bone graft for restoration of length. Foot Ankle Int 2000;21(4):297–330.
11. Treadwell J. First Metatarsophalangeal joint arthrodesis; what is the best fixation option? Clin Podiatr Med Surg 2013;30:327–49.
12. Moon J, McGlamry M. First metatarsophalangeal joint arthrodesis: current fixation options. Clin Podiatr Med Surg 2011;28:405–19.
13. Hunt KJ, Ellington JK, Anderson RB. Locked versus nonlocked plate fixation for hallux MTP arthrodesis. Foot Ankle Int 2011;32:704–9.
14. Doty J, Coughlin M, Hirose C, et al. Hallux metatarsophalangeal joint arthrodesis with a hybrid locking plate and a plantar neutralization screw: a prospective study. Foot Ankle Int 2013;34(11):1535–40.
15. Mann JJ, Moon JL, Brosky TA. Low-profile titanium plate construct for early weightbearing with first metatarsophalangeal joint arthrodesis. J Foot Ankle Surg 2013;52:460–4.
16. Usuelli F, Tamini F, Maccario C, et al. Bone-block arthrodesis procedure in failures of first metatarsophalangeal joint replacement. Foot Ankle Surg 2017;23:163–7.

The Role of Lesser Metatarsophalangeal Joint Arthrodesis for Revision Surgery

Sean T. Grambart, DPM[a,b,*], Nephi E.H. Jones, DPM, PGY2[b]

KEYWORDS

- Crossover toe • Hammertoe • Arthrodesis • Revision surgery

KEY POINTS

- Lesser metatarsophalangeal joint arthrodesis, although not common, provides a good option for revision surgery for a failed hammertoe.
- A stable fixation construct provides an optimal healing environment.
- Optimal positioning of the arthrodesis site will depend heavily on patient postoperative expectations.

INTRODUCTION

Hammertoe surgery is one of the most common procedures performed by foot and ankle surgeons. There are a variety of surgical techniques and implants that can be used to correct a hammertoe. Although the most patients do well, there is a subset of patients who have poor outcomes and unpredictable results.[1–10] Failure of the initial surgery may result in chronic swelling, scar tissue, lack of toe purchase, stiffness, and the inability to wear shoes. When these poor outcomes occur and affect the patient's quality of life, this may require revision surgery.

In the authors' experience, patients who require multiple procedures on lesser digits have increased swelling and scar tissue, which further complicate the recovery and decreases the success rates. Often these patients are looking for a "one-and-done" procedure. Amputation of the toe or a partial ray amputation is an option, but for many patients this is not an acceptable alternative. For patients who refuse amputation unless absolutely necessary, a viable option to consider is lesser metatarsophalangeal joint (MTPJ) arthrodesis. The purpose of this article is to review the literature on the fusion and the surgical technique.

^a Des Moines University, College of Podiatric Medicine and Surgery, 3200 Grand Avenue, Des Moines, IA 50312, USA; ^b Unitypoint Health - Iowa Methodist Medical Center, 1200 Pleasant Street, Des Moines, IA 50309, USA
* Corresponding author. Des Moines University, College of Podiatric Medicine and Surgery, 3200 Grand Avenue, Des Moines, IA 50312.
E-mail address: Sean.Grambart@dmu.edu

Clin Podiatr Med Surg 37 (2020) 433–445
https://doi.org/10.1016/j.cpm.2020.03.006
0891-8422/20/© 2020 Elsevier Inc. All rights reserved.

CURRENT LITERATURE

When discussing lesser MTPJ arthrodesis, there are a limited number of published papers directly related to the topic for primary or revision hammertoe surgery. Currently, the most common surgical options for patients with primary hammertoe deformities with and without MTPJ pathologic condition and failed hammertoe procedures include soft tissue realignment, metatarsal osteotomy, resection arthroplasty, plantar plate repair, and amputation.[1–8,10–19] In retrospect, there has been skepticism in the foot and ankle community about the utility or longevity of lesser MTPJ arthrodesis because many think it is not well tolerated, and some advocate that it should not be undertaken. There is also concern that isolated second MTPJ fusions would fare poorly because of high biomechanical forces on this joint during ambulation.

One of the first published papers on lesser MTPJ arthrodesis was performed by Karlock[20] evaluating second MTPJ arthrodesis in combination with varying first MTPJ procedures for severe crossover hammertoe deformities. The results showed 10 of 11 (91%) achieved radiographic union and excellent clinical results at 19 months. He concluded that this surgical procedure was a direct alternative to amputation and a viable option for severe crossover hammertoe deformities and recommended this in patients with a severely rigid deformity with low ambulation demands.

Hollawell and colleagues[21] reported a case series reviewing 4 patients with 5 lesser MTPJ arthrodeses to address varying causes of lesser MTPJ deformity. They reported that all had risk factors for recurrence and suboptimal or undesirable outcomes if only soft tissue or other osseous procedures were performed instead of arthrodesis. Their reported results were radiographic and clinical union of all 4 patients with no recurrence of deformity at 21 months. They concluded that lesser MTPJ arthrodesis should be reserved for severe, recalcitrant deformities but is a very viable option.

Hirose and colleagues[1] published a case review on 5 patients undergoing concomitant first and second MTPJ arthrodesis for intractable second MTPJ pain. They reported collective AOFAS (American Orthopaedic Foot and Ankle Society) scores increased from 36.8 preoperatively to 78.1 postoperatively and visual analogue scale pain score decreased from 6.8 preoperatively to 1.1 postoperatively. They achieved radiographic and clinical union by 3 months in all patients and had no recurrent deformities over 2.4 years. They impart concern for failure of the lesser MTPJ arthrodesis because of a high degree of force during weight-bearing when this is performed as an isolated procedure and advocated arthrodesis of the first MTPJ as well.

Jeffries and colleagues[22] published a surgical technique paper for multiple MTPJ arthrodesis in the rheumatoid foot as an alternative to the traditional first MPJ arthrodesis with pan metatarsal head resection. They conclude that this procedure may serve as a long-lasting deformity correction for the rheumatoid foot; however, they did not report the clinical results of the paper.

To date, the highest level of clinical evidence related to this topic (level 3) was undertaken by Joseph and colleagues[23] in a retrospective analysis of 31 lesser MTPJ arthrodeses performed by 3 different surgeons as an option for hammertoe pathologic condition, namely MTPJ instability owing to plantar plate pathologic condition. They reported that of the 31 lesser MTPJ fusions, none resulted in a floating toe, and they suggest that concomitant tendon transfer or plantar plate repair was unnecessary. They achieved clinical union at an average of 10 weeks and radiographic union at an average of 8.6 weeks. They also reported that all patients returned to unrestricted activity and shoe gear without the need for orthotics or orthopedic shoes. The pain associated with the preoperative deformity was significantly reduced after fusion at a mean follow-up of 26 months. The patients did not have limitation of shoe gear and did not require the use of orthotics. Again, these investigators suggest that lesser MTPJ arthrodesis is a viable option for complex hammertoe deformities.

Surgical Technique

In the authors' opinion, the indications for a second MTPJ arthrodesis are very limited. These indications include revisional hammertoe/crossover toe surgery in which there has been failure of soft tissue rebalancing procedures and osseous procedures along the MTPJ, significant bone destruction of the metatarsal head, severe rigid deformities of the MTPJs, or degenerative changes of the MTPJ that has failed conservative treatment. The authors consider this procedure a salvage procedure for revision of failed hammertoe in lieu of an amputation. Before the surgery, the authors recommend the patient tape the toe in for at least 1 week to give them some idea of what a lesser MTPJ arthrodesis will feel like (**Fig. 1**).

Case 1

The patient is a 54-year-old woman who presented after previous hammertoe surgery on the second toe consisting of a second proximal interphalangeal joint arthrodesis and distal second metatarsal osteotomy. The metatarsal osteotomy developed an avascular necrosis and subsequent destruction of the head of the metatarsal (**Figs. 2 and 3**). The patient had limitations of shoe gear because of the elevation of the toe, pain with activities, and issues with the appearance of the toe. Options were discussed, including partial ray resection and bone-block distraction arthrodesis. She elected to proceed with distraction arthrodesis.

The procedure is performed as an outpatient procedure typically with the use of a general anesthetic. Thigh tourniquet is used, and often an ipsilateral bump is placed under the hip to help internally rotate the lower limb to provide ideal exposure to the arthrodesis site. A linear or curvilinear incision is made beginning at the junction of the proximal-middle third of the metatarsal and extending distally to the proximal interphalangeal joint of the toe. In many cases, there has been a previous procedure performed at the proximal interphalangeal joint and/or MTPJ, and the surgeon needs to be aware of any retained surgical implants. Deepening Full-thickness dissection should be performed as the incision is deepened (**Fig. 4**). Expect to see some significant scar tissue with entrapment of the extensor tendons. As the metatarsal, proximal phalanx, and joint are exposed, it is imperative to keep the no. 15 blade up against the bone in order to prevent any damage to the vascular structures along the toe. The scar tissue from previous surgeries can entrap the vascular structures as well, which can alter the course of the vessels. Joint preparation is performed with removal of any remaining cartilage using curettage resection or planal resection with a saw (**Fig. 5**). The authors prefer to avoid the use of reamers in this joint because of the fragile nature and limited size of the bone. The authors' preferred method of cartilage resection is curettage in order to preserve some strength of the subchondral bone and adjacent cortices. However, in this case, planal resection was done because of the use of an allograft bone block. The adjacent arthrodesis sites are then fenestrated with a small K-wire or drill bit. In this case, the tourniquet was deflated in order to ensure adequate blood supply to the bone along the second metatarsal given the patient's previous history of avascular necrosis. The allograft selected was an ulnar graft. The graft was placed in the arthrodesis site, and the toe was positioned (**Fig. 6**).

Alignment of the toe on the metatarsal can be a difficult decision. Patient expectations and activities should be discussed in detail preoperatively to help decide the optimal position for the patient. In the sagittal place, the authors have found that most men prefer the toe to purchase the ground, whereas women who like to wear

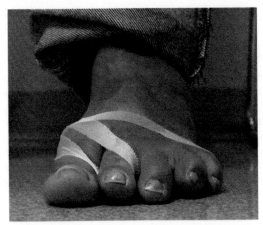

Fig. 1. Before the surgery, the patient tapes the toe 23 hours per day to see if she can tolerate the toe fixed in the anticipated position of the arthrodesis.

shoes with a small heel prefer the toe just slightly off the ground by 1 to 2 mm. If the toe is dorsiflexed too much, the third toe can start to drift into an adductovarus position and ride under the second toe. Transverse plane position will be based on alignment of the hallux and third toe. With a stable positioned hallux, the ideal transverse plane

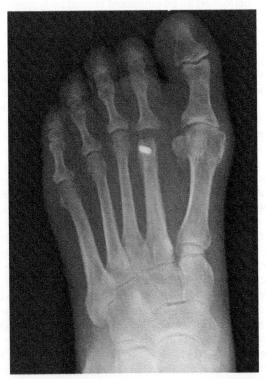

Fig. 2. Preoperative anteroposterior (AP) radiograph shows bone destruction along the second metatarsal.

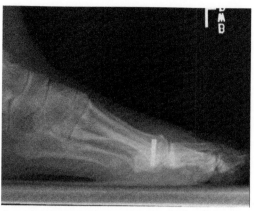

Fig. 3. Preoperative lateral radiograph with elevation of the second toe.

alignment of the second toe is parallel to the hallux. Frontal plane position uses the nail plate/bed. The use of a flat surface intraoperatively is useful with position of the toe similar to how it is used for position of a first MTPJ arthrodesis.

Plate fixation was selected. These plates may need some contouring in order to fit the optimal position of the toe. The authors typically start with a 0° plate and bend as needed. The ultimate goal of the plate is a minimum of 2 screws into the proximal phalanx and a minimum of 2 screws into the metatarsal. Once the plate has been properly contoured, the authors screw the plate into position on the metatarsal typically with a combination of locking and nonlocking screws. Once alignment is confirmed, the plate is fixated on the proximal phalanx with locking screws (**Fig. 7**). Layered closure is

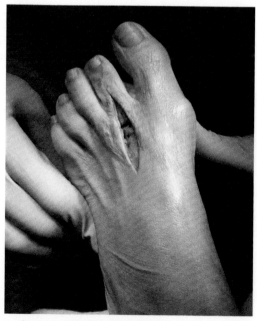

Fig. 4. Linear incision along the dorsal second MTPJ.

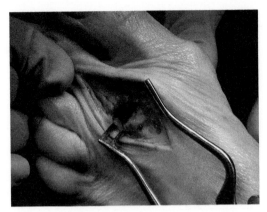

Fig. 5. Preparation of the arthrodesis sites.

performed, and a dry sterile dressing is applied with a posterior splint. Before waking the patient up, the tourniquet is dropped to make sure there is no vascular compromise to the toe. The authors normally do not advance the diet of the patient or apply ice or elevation in the recovery area until they have confirmed the return of adequate blood flow. Postoperative protocol is a non-weight-bearing splint for 10 to 14 days followed by a non-weight-bearing boot for 2 weeks. At the 4-week postoperative visit, radiographs are obtained. If there is adequate healing of the arthrodesis site at that time, then the patient is allowed to weight bear in the boot as tolerated for an additional 4 weeks. At 8-weeks postoperatively, if the radiographs are stable, then they can start to advance into shoes. The authors do recommend limiting the start of exercising for at least 4 more weeks. The patient is normally instructed to follow up in 6 months (**Figs. 8–10**).

Case 2
The patient is a 67-year-old retired nurse with significant toe deformities causing pain and limitation with shoe gear. She has had previous surgery to the first and fifth

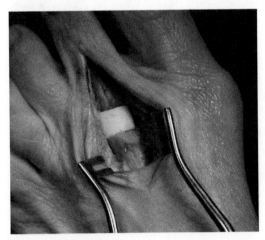

Fig. 6. Placement of the ulnar allograft.

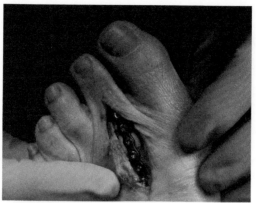

Fig. 7. Plate fixation of the graft and the arthrodesis site.

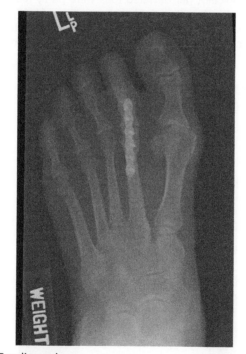

Fig. 8. Six-month AP radiograph.

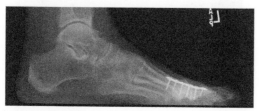

Fig. 9. Six-month lateral radiograph.

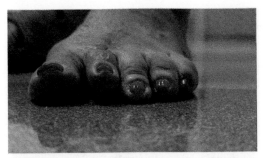

Fig. 10. Postoperative view shows the second toe slightly elevated owing to the patient wanting to wear a shoe with a 1- to 2-inch heel at times.

metatarsals and the second and third hammertoes several years before presenting to the authors' office. Clinically, her deviated toes were partly reducible. Radiographs confirmed extensive deformity with arthritic changes (**Figs. 11–13**). She elected to proceed with lesser MTPJ arthrodesis of the second, third, and fourth MTPJs. The surgical procedure was similar to the case discussed above. Three well-spaced-out

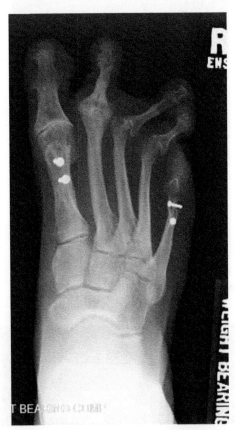

Fig. 11. Preoperative AP radiograph indicating the deformities and arthritic changes.

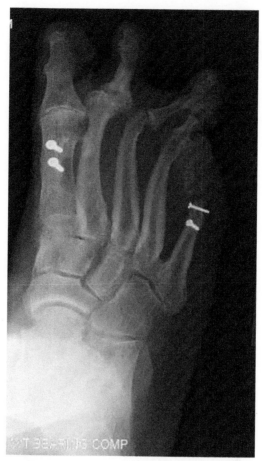

Fig. 12. Preoperative oblique radiograph.

longitudinal incisions were placed on the dorsal surface. Pin fixation was chosen on the fourth toe in order to prevent extensive soft tissue stripping in order for plate fixation. The postoperative protocol was discussed as above. The pin was removed from the fourth toe at 8 weeks postoperatively. Radiographs at 6 months postoperatively are shown in **Figs. 14** and **15**.

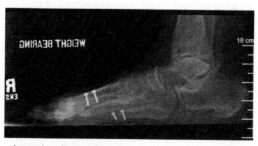

Fig. 13. Preoperative lateral radiograph.

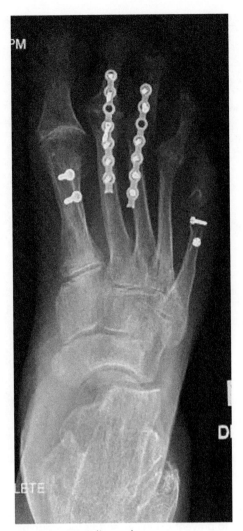

Fig. 14. Six-month postoperative AP radiograph.

Surgical Discussion Points

- If the patient has a bunion deformity, then correction of the bunion should be performed. In these cases, the authors typically recommend an arthrodesis of the first MTPJ for the bunion correction.
- The authors have used compression screws with plate fixation as well. If a compression screw is used, one should make sure there is adequate distance of the start of the guide wire and the MTPJ. If it is too close to the joint, as the compression screw is inserted, it can crack the cortex of the proximal phalanx. The authors have not seen any difference in starting the screw from the medial or lateral aspect of the proximal phalanx. Before placement of the compression screw, the authors like to position the dorsal plate.

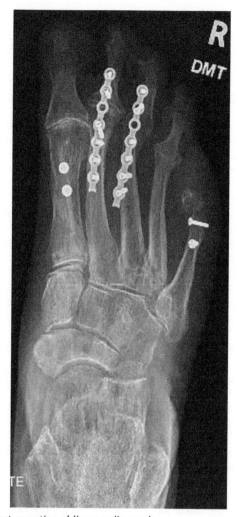

Fig. 15. Six-month postoperative oblique radiograph.

SUMMARY

The authors' have seen good success with lesser MTPJ arthrodesis with severe deformities and when used for salvage procedures instead of an amputation. With the limited amount of published evidence on this subject, there is a need to perform more rigorous investigation with larger study groups and longer outcome results. With that being said, lesser MTPJ arthrodesis seems to be a very viable and reasonable option for either revision hammertoe surgeries or as a primary surgical option for hammertoe correction in the appropriate patient.

DISCLOSURE

S.T. Grambart: Partner BESPA Global. No conflicts with the material within this article.

REFERENCES

1. Hirose CB, Gamboa JT, Coughlin MJ. Concomitant first and second metatarsophalangeal arthrodesis for intractable second metatarsophalangeal joint pain. Foot Ankle Int 2014;35(8):825–8.
2. Myerson MS, Jung HG. The role of toe flexor-to-extensor transfer in correcting metatarsophalangeal joint instability of the second toe. Foot Ankle Int 2005; 26(9):675–9.
3. Saltzman CL, Johnson KA, Donnelly RE. Surgical treatment for mild deformities of the rheumatoid forefoot by partial phalangectomy and syndactylization. Foot Ankle 1993;14(6):325–9.
4. Cook JJ, Johnson LJ, Cook EA. Anatomic reconstruction versus traditional rebalancing in lesser metatarsophalangeal joint reconstruction. J Foot Ankle Surg 2018;57(3):509–13.
5. Boffeli TJ, Thompson JC, Tabatt JA. Two-pin fixation of proximal interphalangeal joint fusion for hammertoe correction. J Foot Ankle Surg 2016;55(3):480–7.
6. Ceccarini P, Ceccarini A, Rinonapoli G, et al. Correction of hammer toe deformity of lateral toes with subtraction osteotomy of the proximal phalanx neck. J Foot Ankle Surg 2015;54(4):601–6.
7. Bouche RT, Heit EJ. Combined plantar plate and hammertoe repair with flexor digitorum longus tendon transfer for chronic, severe sagittal plane instability of the lesser metatarsophalangeal joints: preliminary observations. J Foot Ankle Surg 2008;47(2):125–37.
8. Solan MC, Davies MS. Revision surgery of the lesser toes. Foot Ankle Clin 2011; 16(4):621–45.
9. Albright RH, Hassan M, Randich J, et al. Risk factors for failure in hammertoe surgery. Foot Ankle Int 2020. 1071100720904931.
10. Myerson MS, Fortin P, Girard P. Use of skin Z-plasty for management of extension contracture in recurrent claw- and hammertoe deformity. Foot Ankle Int 1994; 15(4):209–12.
11. Ellis SJ, Young E, Endo Y, et al. Correction of multiplanar deformity of the second toe with metatarsophalangeal release and extensor brevis reconstruction. Foot Ankle Int 2013;34(6):792–9.
12. Ford LA, Collins KB, Christensen JC. Stabilization of the subluxed second metatarsophalangeal joint: flexor tendon transfer versus primary repair of the plantar plate. J Foot Ankle Surg 1998;37(3):217–22.
13. Johansen JK, Jordan M, Thomas M. Clinical and radiological outcomes after Weil osteotomy compared to distal metatarsal metaphyseal osteotomy in the treatment of metatarsalgia–a prospective study. Foot Ankle Surg 2019;25(4):488–94.
14. Rivero-Santana A, Perestelo-Perez L, Garces G, et al. Clinical effectiveness and safety of Weil's osteotomy and distal metatarsal mini-invasive osteotomy (DMMO) in the treatment of metatarsalgia: a systematic review. Foot Ankle Surg 2019; 25(5):565–70.
15. Yeo NE, Loh B, Chen JY, et al. Comparison of early outcome of Weil osteotomy and distal metatarsal mini-invasive osteotomy for lesser toe metatarsalgia. J Orthop Surg (Hong Kong) 2016;24(3):350–3.
16. Trask DJ, Ledoux WR, Whittaker EC, et al. Second metatarsal osteotomies for metatarsalgia: a robotic cadaveric study of the effect of osteotomy plane and metatarsal shortening on plantar pressure. J Orthop Res 2014;32(3):385–93.
17. Winson IG, Rawlinson J, Broughton NS. Treatment of metatarsalgia by sliding distal metatarsal osteotomy. Foot Ankle 1988;9(1):2–6.

18. Reikeras O. Metatarsal osteotomy for relief of metatarsalgia. Arch Orthop Trauma Surg 1983;101(3):177–8.
19. Helal B. Metatarsal osteotomy for metatarsalgia. J Bone Joint Surg Br 1975;57(2): 187–92.
20. Karlock LG. Second metatarsophalangeal joint fusion: a new technique for cross-over hammertoe deformity. A preliminary report. J Foot Ankle Surg 2003;42(4): 178–82.
21. Hollawell SM, Kane BJ, Paternina JP, et al. Lesser metatarsophalangeal joint pathology addressed with arthrodesis: a case series. J Foot Ankle Surg 2019;58(2): 387–91.
22. Jeffries LC, Rodriguez RH, Stapleton JJ, et al. Pan-metatarsophalangeal joint arthrodesis for the severe rheumatoid forefoot deformity. Clin Podiatr Med Surg 2009;26(1):149–57.
23. Joseph R, Schroeder K, Greenberg M. A retrospective analysis of lesser metatarsophalangeal joint fusion as a treatment option for hammertoe pathology associated with metatarsophalangeal joint instability. J Foot Ankle Surg 2012;51(1): 57–62.

Trephine Procedure for Revision Tarsometatarsal Arthrodesis Nonunion

Sean T. Grambart, DPM[a,b,*], Eric R. Reese, DPM[b]

KEYWORDS

- Lisfranc • Tarsometatarsal • Arthrodesis • Revision surgery

KEY POINTS

- Trephine technique provides an excellent option for revision tarsometatarsal joint arthrodesis.
- A stable fixation construct provides an optimal healing environment.
- Maintaining a 1-mm cortical edge around the medial, lateral, and plantar cortex aids in stability.

INTRODUCTION

Midfoot arthritis is a common condition treated by foot and ankle surgeons. Although this procedure is commonly performed, there is limited literature on the tarsometatarsal arthritis and treatment outcomes.[1–9] The causes of midfoot arthritis are numerous including post-traumatic, osteoarthritis caused by obesity or biomechanical deformities, or inflammatory arthritis (**Fig. 1**). Common patient complaints include aching pain with activity and burning pain along the dorsal foot. Clinical signs of midfoot arthritis include dorsal osteophytes, or pain with isolated movement of the tarsometatarsal joint. Radiographs generally show osteophyte formation and joint space narrowing.

Initial treatment is usually conservative with orthotics, rocker bottom shoes, intra-articular steroids, or combination therapy. When conservative treatment fails, arthrodesis is indicated. Unfortunately, because of the unique anatomy, traditional preparation of the joints involves shortening of bony structures and extensive dissection and releasing adjacent articulations, ligaments, and other soft tissue structures.

[a] Des Moines University, College of Podiatric Medicine and Surgery, 3200 Grand Avenue, Des Moines, IA 50312, USA; [b] Unitypoint Health - Iowa Methodist Medical Center, 1200 Pleasant Street, Des Moines, IA 50309, USA
* Corresponding author. Des Moines University, College of Podiatric Medicine and Surgery, 3200 Grand Avenue, Des Moines, IA 50312.
E-mail address: Sean.Grambart@dmu.edu

Clin Podiatr Med Surg 37 (2020) 447–461
https://doi.org/10.1016/j.cpm.2020.03.001
0891-8422/20/© 2020 Elsevier Inc. All rights reserved.

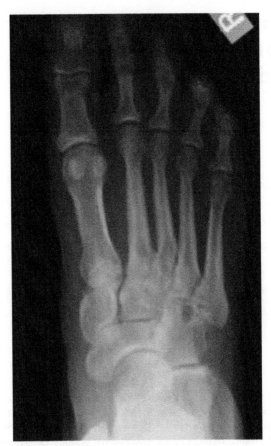

Fig. 1. Anteroposterior radiograph of tarsometatarsal arthritis.

Current literature is somewhat lacking regarding arthrodesis rates specific to mid-foot fusions with the trephine technique. Ryan and colleagues[10] performed a cadaveric study to aid in the process of joint preparation by looking at average depth of the Lisfranc joint. After studying 51 specimens they determined the average depth of the first metatarsal-cuneiform joint to be 32.3 mm, the second metatarsal-cuneiform joint to be 26.9 mm, and the third metatarsal-cuneiform joint to be 23.6 mm. They also observed a positive correlation with length of the foot relative to the depth of the joints. Based on these measurements some individuals recommend taking a shorter plug to preserve the plantar cortex for additional stabilization.

In regard to Lisfranc arthrodesis rates using traditional methods of joint preparation and fixation (curettage with plates or screws), Buda and colleagues[1] demonstrated an overall 11.4% nonunion rate while retrospectively reviewing 189 joints. Higher rates of nonunion were associated with plate fixation with all screws through the plate, smoking perioperatively, and nonanatomic realignment. One reason curettage could lead to higher nonunion rates could be because of reasons found in a cadaveric study by Johnson and coworkers.[11] Histologic review of all cadaveric specimens prepared for arthrodesis demonstrated a residual layer of calcified cartilage overlying the subchondral plate. They concluded this barrier may interfere with bony consolidation of the arthrodesis site.

Although no large high-quality studies are known to the authors, this nonunion rate can be compared with smaller studies and case reports. Withey and colleagues[12] described his technique for trephine arthrodesis of the midfoot in 2014 and experienced no nonunions. Filiatrault and Banks[13] have used a similar trephine technique of multiple joints in the foot and ankle. Their review of 22 joints of the tarsometatarsal joints, naviculocuneiform joint, subtalar joint, and ankle joint revealed a 95% successful arthrodesis rate. Teasdall and colleagues[14] reported on three cases of midfoot arthrodesis with 100% union rate. Although evidence regarding arthrodesis rates with the trephine plug is limited, there is evidence that midfoot arthrodesis rates are enhanced with autogenous grafting.[1]

Trephine arthrodesis has been described in the literature for several years. Trephines initially were developed in the 1940s and were predominantly used in spinal surgery.[15] The use of trephine arthrodesis has been described in arthrodesis of the foot and ankle literature with good results since the early 1990s.[16] This is particularly true in instances when the arthritic joints are in good alignment and an in situ arthrodesis can be performed. Multiple trephine techniques have been described including complete or partial resection of the joint surfaces, use of iliac crest or calcaneal graft, or rotating the internal segment 90° without supplemental grafting. Traditionally fixation of the graft segment was not used; however, more recently the dowel graft has been fixated with staples, plates, or screws, which is believed to provide better compression and fixation of the graft, and ultimately lower nonunion and complication rates.

Not only has the trephine technique been proven, it is also noted the technique to harvest calcaneal bone graft described by Roukis[17] has proven to be technically easy and safe. This technique is reproducible and has a low incidence of complications including wound dehiscence, calcaneal fracture, and donor site morbidity.[12]

In arthritic joints that require realignment, the trephine approach is difficult and more traditional planal resections arthrodesis offer the surgeon a better choice (**Figs. 2 and 3**).[13] However, when the trephine approach is indicated, it offers many advantages including minimal soft tissue dissection, quicker joint preparation, and the minimal shortening of the arthrodesis site. Given these advantages, the authors have found the trephine approach to be the procedure of choice in correction of a nonunion.

SURGICAL TECHNIQUE

The authors' preferred surgical procedure for a revision of a nonunion lesser tarsometatarsal is a trephine approach for the nonunion preparation site and the autograft harvest site. The procedure is performed either as an inpatient-overnight stay or outpatient procedure. This is typically performed with the use of a general anesthetic. A thigh tourniquet is used and often an ipsilateral bump is placed under the hip to help internally rotate the lower limb to provide ideal exposure to the dorsal midfoot area.

With initial surgery for second and third tarsometatarsal arthrodesis, we prefer a single incision to expose both joints. However, in cases of revision surgery, we recommend using the previous incision or incisions that were used. Scar tissue is commonly present that may entrap some of the branches of the intermediate dorsal cutaneous nerve and the extensor tendons. With dissection, the goal is to attempt to raise this area of entrapment as a flap of tissue to aid in closure and avoid iatrogenic damage to these tendon and nerves. Some scar tissue can be resected along the tendons, but only if it will not be a detriment to skin closure. As the dissection is deepened, care must be taken to stay on the medial aspect of the second

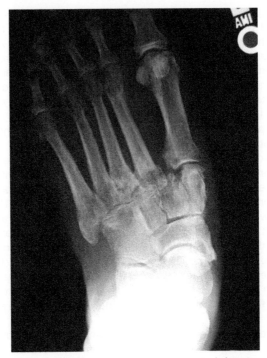

Fig. 2. Anteroposterior radiograph of midfoot arthritis with deformity.

tarsometatarsal revision site and not dissect into the first interspace near the deep plantar artery and deep peroneal nerve.

If there is hardware along the nonunion, this needs to be removed. We recommend leaving any fractured screws unless they are easily visualized and can be removed without the need for overzealous removal of bone. The nonunion sites are difficult to visualize because of the fibrous tissue and nature of the small size of the joints. A ronguer is used to gently remove the very dorsal fibrous tissue to aid in the visualization of the nonunion sites. Once the fibrous tissue has been removed, the surgeon should make an attempt to move the tarsometatarsal nonunion sites to identify proper

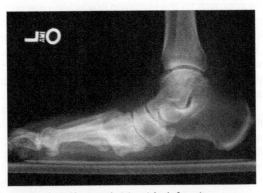

Fig. 3. Lateral radiograph of midfoot arthritis with deformity.

location of the joints. With the aid of intraoperative fluoroscopy, a freer or Kirschner wire can also help to identify the nonunion sites. One of the advantages of the trephine technique is that it is performed without having to dissect a large amount to soft tissue around the bone, so all that needs to be done is to identify the nonunion site.

There are multiple systems that are available with trephine reamers including foot and ankle sets and some anterior cruciate ligament reamer sets. Starting with the second tarsometatarsal, a guide pin from the reamer set is placed within the nonunion site (**Fig. 4**). A special point of emphasis is that the pin needs to be in the center of the nonunion site. When placing the guide pin for the reamer, the orientation needs to be more of a dorsal-lateral to plantar-medial direction compared with the guide pin of the second tarsometatarsal given the natural "Roman-arch" shape of the Lisfranc area. Once the guide pin is placed, confirmation of the proper placement is achieved by using fluoroscopy with the center ray following the line of the pin (**Fig. 5**). Once the placement of the pin is confirmed, a reamer is selected. Normally for the second tarsometatarsal, the reamer is usually 8.5 or 9.5 mm in diameter (**Fig. 6**). These reamers are designed to remove the section of bone. Resection should remove all of the fibrous tissue and dysvascular bone. The remaining bone should be ideal with the bone having a rich blood supply to support the healing of the graft and nonunion site. The key is to resect as much of the nonunion site as possible while trying to keep approximately 1 mm along the outer diameter to try to preserve the medial, lateral, and plantar cortices. Preserving the medial and lateral cortices aids in the stability of the arthrodesis sites (**Fig. 7**). Preserving the plantar cortex not only aids to stability but also prevents the graft from migrating plantarly (**Fig. 8**). The foot and ankle reamer set that the authors use have a maximum depth of 25 mm. Because the average depth of the second tarsometatarsal joint is 26.9 mm, the plantar cortex is rarely disrupted. More care must be used with the third tarsometatarsal joint because the average depth of the third tarsometatarsal joint is 23.6 mm. The typical reamer diameter used for the third tarsometatarsal joint is 8.5 mm (**Fig. 9**).

There are multiple options for sites to harvest the autograft, but the authors prefer the calcaneus because it is readily accessible, and it does not alter the recovery process. A linear incision is made along the lateral aspect of the calcaneus. This location

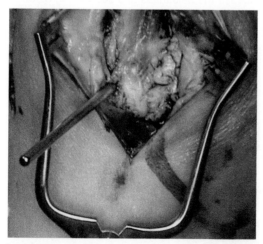

Fig. 4. Placement of the trephine guidewire along the center of the second tarsometatarsal joint.

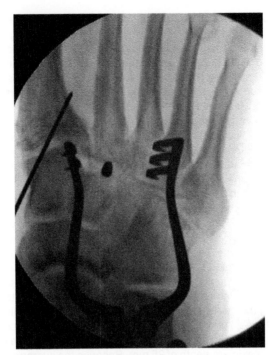

Fig. 5. Intraoperative fluoroscopy confirmation of the guide pin.

should be posterior to the course of the sural nerve. The dissection is deepened to expose the lateral aspect of the calcaneus. To harvest the graft, the same reamers are used (**Fig. 10**). The harvest of the grafts can either be positioned superior and inferior or posterior to anterior (**Figs. 11** and **12**). We recommend trying to leave a bone bridge between the harvest sites for stability. After the autografts are harvested, the harvest sites are back filled with cancellous bone chips to serve as a scaffolding for healing (**Fig. 13**). Because the calcaneus has such a rich blood supply, single layer

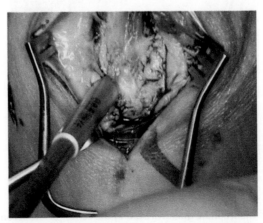

Fig. 6. Trephine placement along the second tarsometatarsal arthrodesis site.

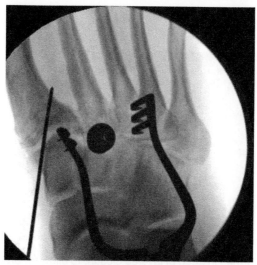

Fig. 7. Intraoperative fluoroscopy confirmation of maintaining the cortices.

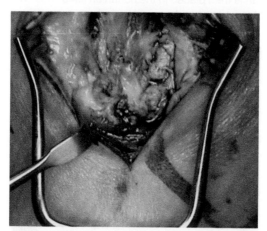

Fig. 8. Resection of the joint surface of the second tarsometatarsal with maintaining plantar cortex.

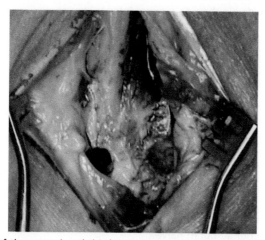

Fig. 9. Resection of the second and third tarsometatarsal arthrodesis sites.

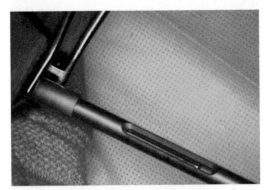

Fig. 10. Trephine removal of the autograft from the lateral cortex of the calcaneus.

skin closure is performed instead of layered closure to allow for drainage of the blood though the incision.

The harvested graft is then placed in the nonunion sites. This should be a "press-fit" fashion. If the plantar cortex has been disrupted, care must be taken to avoid the

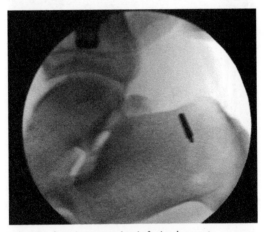

Fig. 11. Trephine guide pin showing superior-inferior harvest.

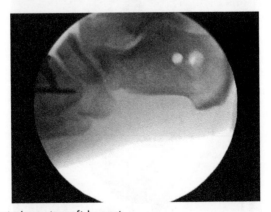

Fig. 12. Anteroposterior autograft harvest.

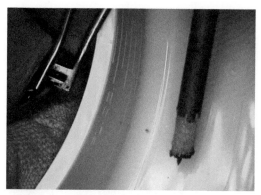

Fig. 13. Calcaneal autograft.

pushing of the graft through plantar cortex (**Figs. 14** and **15**). Fixation is placed over the top of the graft and nonunion sites. The authors have used a variety of fixation constructs. Initially, locking plate constructs with a combination of locking and nonlocking screws were used (**Fig. 16**). If this type of fixation is selected, once the plate is properly positioned, the authors technique involves first using nonlocking screws in a hole

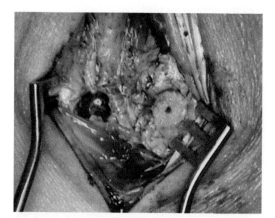

Fig. 14. Press-fit autograft into the third tarsometatarsal arthrodesis site.

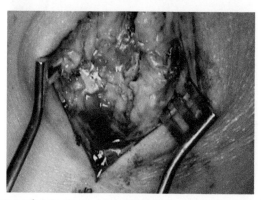

Fig. 15. Press-fit autograft into the second and third tarsometatarsal arthrodesis site.

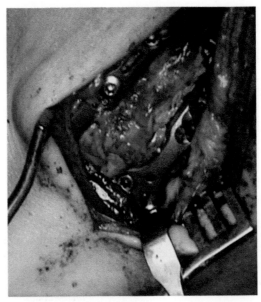

Fig. 16. Plate fixation of the arthrodesis sites.

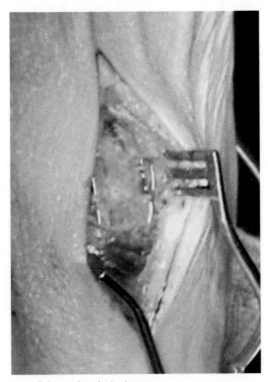

Fig. 17. Staple fixation of the arthrodesis sites.

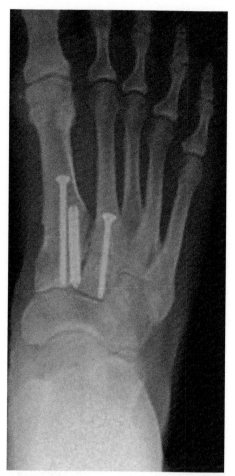

Fig. 18. Anteroposterior radiograph showing nonunion second tarsometatarsal arthrodesis site.

distal to the arthrodesis site and one proximal to the arthrodesis site to make sure the plate is against the bone. Locking screws can then be used in the remaining holes. More recently, the authors preferred method of fixation is nitinol staples (**Fig. 17**). The staples offer the advantages of less soft tissue dissection and quicker insertion. Once the hardware has been placed, intraoperative fluoroscopy is used to confirm the alignment of the hardware. Layered closure is performed, and a dry sterile dressing is applied with a posterior splint.

Postoperative protocol is nonweightbearing splint for 10 to 14 days followed by a nonweightbearing boot for 2 weeks. At the 4-week postoperative visit, radiographs are obtained. If there is adequate healing of the arthrodesis site at that time, then the patient is allowed to begin weightbearing in the boot as tolerated for an additional 4 weeks. At 8 weeks postoperative, if the radiographs are stable, then they can start advance into shoes. The authors do recommend limiting the start of exercising for at least 4 more weeks. Physical therapy is used to aid in advancement of activities. The patient is normally instructed to follow-up in 6 months.

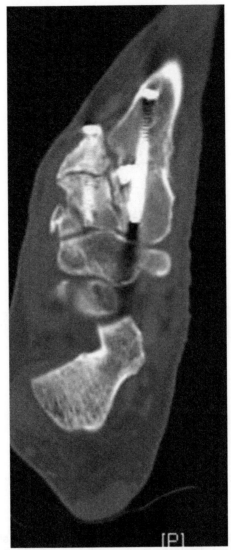

Fig. 19. Computed tomography imaging confirming nonunion second tarsometatarsal arthrodesis site.

CASE 1

This is a 55-year-old woman with a history of a first and second tarsometatarsal arthrodesis performed 1 year prior. She had continued pain along the second tarso-metatarsal arthrodesis site. Radiographs reveal successful arthrodesis of the first tar-sometatarsal arthrodesis site, whereas radiographs and computed tomography scans show nonunion of the second tarsometatarsal arthrodesis site (**Figs. 18** and **19**). Attempted conservative treatment was prolonged immobilization and bone stimulator for 3 months without alleviating the pain. Patient elected to proceed with revision arthrodesis using the trephine method described previously. Imaging shows success-ful healing of the arthrodesis site (**Figs. 20** and **21**).

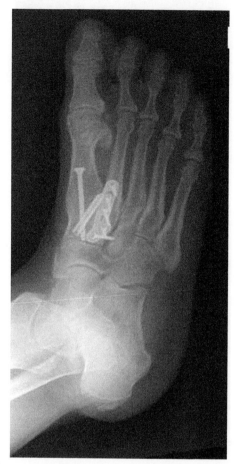

Fig. 20. Six-month oblique radiograph showing healing of the revision site.

KEY SURGICAL POINTS

- Resect as much of the nonunion site as possible while trying to keep approximately 1 mm along the outer diameter to try to preserve the medial, lateral, and plantar cortices. Preserving the medial and lateral cortices aids in the stability of the arthrodesis sites.
- Preserving the plantar cortex not only aids to stability but also prevents the graft from migrating plantarly.
- The average depth of the second tarsometatarsal joint is 26.9 mm. The average depth of the third tarsometatarsal joint is 23.6 mm.[10]
- After the autografts are harvested, the harvest sites are back filled with cancellous bone chips to serve as a scaffolding for healing (**Fig. 22**).

DISCLOSURE

S.T. Grambart is a Partner at BESPA Global. No conflicts with the material within this article.

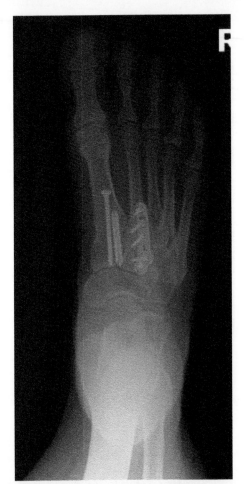

Fig. 21. Six-month anteroposterior radiograph showing healing of the revision site.

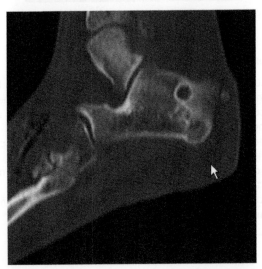

Fig. 22. Computed tomography scan showing healing of the harvest site inferiorly that was filled with cancellous chips. Superior site was not and shows minimal healing.

REFERENCES

1. Buda M, Hagemeijer NC, Kink S, et al. Effect of fixation type and bone graft on tarsometatarsal fusion. Foot Ankle Int 2018;39(12):1394–402.
2. Ebalard M, Le Henaff G, Sigonney G, et al. Risk of osteoarthritis secondary to partial or total arthrodesis of the subtalar and midtarsal joints after a minimum follow-up of 10 years. Orthop Traumatol Surg Res 2014;100(4 Suppl):S231–7.
3. Gougoulias N, Lampridis V. Midfoot arthrodesis. Foot Ankle Surg 2016;22(1): 17–25.
4. Jung HG, Myerson MS, Schon LC. Spectrum of operative treatments and clinical outcomes for atraumatic osteoarthritis of the tarsometatarsal joints. Foot Ankle Int 2007;28(4):482–9.
5. Komenda GA, Myerson MS, Biddinger KR. Results of arthrodesis of the tarsometatarsal joints after traumatic injury. J Bone Joint Surg Am 1996;78(11):1665–76.
6. Sayeed SA, Khan FA, Turner NS 3rd, et al. Midfoot arthritis. Am J Orthop (Belle Mead NJ) 2008;37(5):251–6.
7. Nemec SA, Habbu RA, Anderson JG, et al. Outcomes following midfoot arthrodesis for primary arthritis. Foot Ankle Int 2011;32(4):355–61.
8. Boffeli TJ, Pfannenstein RR, Thompson JC. Combined medial column primary arthrodesis, middle column open reduction internal fixation, and lateral column pinning for treatment of Lisfranc fracture-dislocation injuries. J Foot Ankle Surg 2014;53(5):657–63.
9. Boffeli TJ, Collier RC, Schnell KR. Combined medial column arthrodesis with open reduction internal fixation of central column for treatment of Lisfranc fracture-dislocation: a review of consecutive cases. J Foot Ankle Surg 2018; 57(6):1059–66.
10. Ryan JD, Timpano ED, Brosky TA 2nd. Average depth of tarsometatarsal joint for trephine arthrodesis. J Foot Ankle Surg 2012;51(2):168–71.
11. Johnson JT, Schuberth JM, Thornton SD, et al. Joint curettage arthrodesis technique in the foot: a histological analysis. J Foot Ankle Surg 2009;48(5):558–64.
12. Withey CJ, Murphy AL, Horner R. Tarsometatarsal joint arthrodesis with trephine joint resection and dowel calcaneal bone graft. J Foot Ankle Surg 2014;53(2): 243–7.
13. Filiatrault AD, Banks AS. Trephine arthrodesis of the foot and ankle: indications, operative technique, and long-term follow-up. J Am Podiatr Med Assoc 2006; 96(3):198–204.
14. Teasdall RD, Johnson KA, Hickman ML. The Rochester bone trephine for small joint arthrodesis in the foot. Foot Ankle 1993;14(7):418–23.
15. Michele AA, Harper TC. A method of spinal fusion by arthrodesis and iliac bone grafts. Mil Surg 1949;104(2):90–4.
16. Johnson JE, Johnson KA. Dowel arthrodesis for degenerative arthritis of the tarsometatarsal (Lisfranc) joints. Foot Ankle 1986;6(5):243–53.
17. Roukis T. A simple technique for harvesting autogenous bone grafts from the calcaneus. Foot Ankle Int 2006;27(11):998–9.

Revision Surgery for Failed Lateral Ankle Stabilization

Sean T. Grambart, DPM[a,b,*], Joseph R. Brown, BS[a]

KEYWORDS

- Lateral ankle instability ● Ankle sprain ● Allograft ● Revision surgery

KEY POINTS

- Allograft lateral ankle ligament anatomic reconstruction seems to be a good option for revision surgery.
- Patients that have failed a previous lateral ankle procedure need to be evaluated for conditions that lead to ligament laxity or biomechanical issues.
- Although allografts avoid donor site complications, they do have the disadvantages of increased cost, availability, and extremely low risk of disease transmission.

INTRODUCTION

Ankle sprains are the most common athletic injury in the United States with a reported prevalence between 30% and 40% of all athletic injuries.[1,2] Most patients who suffer a lateral ankle sprain improve with conservative treatment. There are a small number of patients that go onto chronic ankle instability that limits their normal activities. In this group of patients in which conservative treatment fails and limitations are still present, surgical intervention is the likely option. Traditionally there are three types of repairs that have been described: (1) anatomic repair, (2) nonanatomic reconstruction, and (3) anatomic reconstruction. Nonanatomic reconstruction has been shown to increase inversion stiffness and is no longer a common procedure.[3] Most anatomic repairs (ie, Brostrom-Gould procedure) have good to excellent outcomes with low revision rates.[1,4–10] A recent systematic review reported a revision rate of 1.2% in a total of 669 Brostrom-Gould procedures.[4] They cited an overly tight reconstruction as the primary reason for revision.

Even with the high success rate with anatomic repairs, there are still failures and revision surgeries are needed. In certain patients, ligament repairs may have certain factors that could lead to the need for a revision surgery. These factors include:

[a] Des Moines University, College of Podiatric Medicine and Surgery, 3200 Grand Avenue, Des Moines, IA 50312, USA; [b] Unitypoint Health - Iowa Methodist Medical Center, 1200 Pleasant Street, Des Moines, IA 50309, USA
* Corresponding author. Des Moines University, College of Podiatric Medicine and Surgery, 3200 Grand Avenue, Des Moines, IA 50312.
E-mail address: Sean.Grambart@dmu.edu

Clin Podiatr Med Surg 37 (2020) 463–473
https://doi.org/10.1016/j.cpm.2020.03.002
0891-8422/20/© 2020 Elsevier Inc. All rights reserved.

inherited connective tissue disorders, generalized ligamentous laxity, biomechanical abnormalities, and poor tissue quality.

ASSOCIATED FACTORS

Ligament laxity represents one of the major risks for failure of the Brostrom-Gould procedure. Inherited connective tissue disorders, such as Marfan syndrome, Ehlers-Danlos syndrome, and osteogenesis imperfecta, are associated with increased joint laxity. The biomechanical properties of anatomic tissues in patients with these connective tissue disorders are decreased[11] and several authors have suggested that autogenous tissue may be unsuitable for stabilization in these patients.[12,13]

Generalized ligamentous laxity has been associated with recurrent ankle instability. Park and colleagues[12] reported that recurrent instability was much more common in patients with generalized ligamentous laxity (23.8%) compared with those without laxity (3.8%) after a Brostrom procedure. The authors concluded that generalized ligamentous laxity is an independent predictor for poor outcomes following a modified Brostrom procedure. Karlsson and colleagues[8] found that direct repair of lateral ligaments in patients with ligamentous laxity yielded poor results and concluded that this may be a contraindication to the procedure. Messer and colleagues[14] reported that all the patients with generalized ligamentous laxity in their study had poor outcomes and overall lower satisfaction scores. Another study found a 6% failure rate in 49 patients undergoing a modified Brostrom procedure. All failures occurred in patients with Beighton scores greater than 4.[15]

The nine-point Beighton scoring system is used to evaluate patients for joint hypermobility.[16] One point is given for each of the following criteria: passive dorsiflexion of the fifth fingers beyond 90°, apposition of the thumbs to the flexor aspects of the forearms, hyperextension of the elbows beyond 10°, hyperextension of the knees beyond 10°, and trunk flexion with the knees straight and palms resting flat on the floor (**Figs. 1** and **2**). A score of greater than 4 is suggestive of generalized joint hypermobility.[12,17]

Biomechanical issues that are not addressed either before the repair or at the time of the repair can also lead to potential failure. Patients with chronic lateral ankle

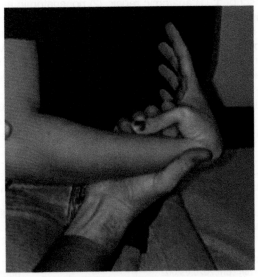

Fig. 1. Thumb to forearm test for ligament laxity.

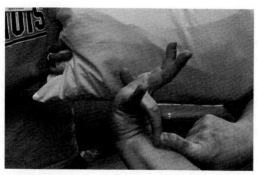

Fig. 2. Extreme ligament laxity.

instability and concomitant cavovarus foot deformity presents a challenge for foot and ankle surgeons (**Fig. 3**). The cavovarus foot is often associated with congenital neuropathies, such as Charcot-Marie-Tooth disease, leading to longstanding muscle imbalances and osseous deformity.[18] Chronic lateral ankle instability is more common in patients with cavovarus foot deformity and is associated with increased failure rates if the underlying cavovarus deformity is not properly addressed.[2,19] O'Neil and Guyton[20] state that hindfoot varus, first ray plantarflexion, and midfoot cavus malalignment deformities can all lead to increased risk of repetitive lateral ankle sprains and early operative failure. Therefore, the cavovarus foot deformity should be corrected at the time of lateral ankle ligamentous repair to prevent failure.[20]

Even patients with a higher body mass index (BMI) may be at increased risk of lateral ankle sprains. Tyler and colleagues[21] followed high school football players over the course of a season and found that overweight athletes are at an increased risk of

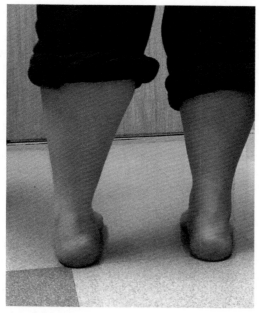

Fig. 3. Varus deformity of the calcaneus.

lateral ankle sprains. Given the higher incidence of ankle sprain, there has been no study in the literature to establish a BMI cutoff to determine when doing a Brostrom would be contraindicated. Park and colleagues[12] found that a BMI greater than 25 was not significantly associated with failure after the modified Brostrom procedure. Additionally, Xu and Lee[22] demonstrated that BMI, sex, and age were not associated with increased failure rates in groups with or without generalized joint laxity.

Timing of the repair does not seem to be a factor that determines success rates. Delayed repair of ruptured lateral ankle ligaments is performed with comparable results to immediate repair.[17,23] Several authors have stated that delayed anatomic repair of lateral ankle ligaments is a viable option, even years after the initial injury.[13,23,24] In a study by Gould and colleagues,[23] they compared their results of patients who received early or late repair. Fifty patients received late repair at a maximum of 13 years, and an average of 2 to 3 years, from the time of initial injury. They achieved similar subjective and functional outcomes compared with patients who had early intervention, and no patients required a revision surgery at final follow-up.

In patients with chronic mechanical instability, the repetitive trauma may lead to associated pathology that can cause pain and limitations. The high prevalence of peroneal tenosynovitis, anterolateral ankle impingement, talar osteochondral lesions, and other pathologies in patients with chronic lateral ankle instability has been demonstrated in multiple studies.[17,25,26] The potential role of these pathologies in poor outcomes following surgery has been brought into question by several authors.[25–27] Choi and colleagues[27] found that the presence of intra-articular lesions can result in poor patient outcomes following lateral ankle ligament repair. They defined a Karlsson-Peterson Ankle Score of less than 90 as an unsatisfactory improvement. In their study, they found that syndesmosis widening was the strongest predictor of an unsatisfactory score. Additional factors that were significantly associated with poor outcomes included osteochondral lesions of the talus and ossicles at the lateral malleolus. Park and colleagues[12] reported that syndesmosis widening is significantly higher in those with generalized ligamentous laxity (13/42; 31%) compared with those without generalized ligamentous laxity (13/157; 8.4%). They also found that generalized ligamentous laxity, syndesmosis widening, osteochondral lesions of the talus, high preoperative talar tilt angle (>15), and high preoperative anterior displacement of the talus (>10 mm) were all significantly associated with clinical failure following the modified Brostrom procedure. In contrast, Okuda and colleagues[26] found focal chondral lesions in 63% of 30 ankles with chronic lateral ankle instability. The postoperative clinical scores were similar between patients with focal chondral lesions and those without lesions. Similarly, Araoye and colleagues[25] found that patients with one or more associated pathologies had similar reoperation rates compared with patients without any associated pathology. Additionally, patients with peroneal pathology had a lower reoperation rate than those without peroneal pathology. The authors note that this could be caused by increased symptoms in these patients leading to them being treated more completely intraoperatively.

ALLOGRAFT LITERATURE

The authors have found that with the surgical approach of addressing the previously mentioned pathologies and performing anatomic reconstruction with allograft can lead to a good and functional outcome. The use of allograft in foot and ankle surgery has been well studied especially for lateral ankle ligament repairs. In a recent review, Diniz and colleagues[28] performed a systematic analysis and found that there is a fair amount of evidence (grade B) in favor of the use of allografts for lateral ankle ligament reconstruction. In 2020, Li and colleagues[29] performed a systematic review of outcomes with the use of allografts for anatomic lateral ankle ligament reconstruction. Six clinical trials with 153 patients found the mean pooled postoperative American Orthopaedic Foot & Ankle Society score was 89.4%, 80% returned to sports, and a there was a 6% risk of recurrent instability. The authors concluded that anatomic lateral ankle reconstruction resulted in significant improvement in function and outcome scores with a low risk of recurrent instability.

AUTHORS' SURGICAL TECHNIQUE

The patient is positioned supine on the operating room table. A bump is placed under the ipsilateral hip to help expose the lateral ankle. If ankle arthroscopy is performed, the bump may be placed after the arthroscopy is complete. A thigh tourniquet is applied. The leg is prepared and draped to make sure the knee is visible to serve as a reference point if needed. All associated procedures (arthroscopy, osseous procedures) are performed before the lateral ankle ligament reconstruction.

A linear incision is made beginning proximal to the tip of the fibula and extending distally toward the anterior process of the calcaneus (**Fig. 4**). This incision is placed slightly more posterior to midline of the fibula not only to help with the evaluation of the peroneal tendons, but also to help better visualize the lateral calcaneus for graft placement.

The incision is deepened with care to protect the intermediate dorsal cutaneous branch off of the superficial peroneal nerve. This typically is retracted medially with minimal tension on the nerve. As the dissection is deepened, the peroneal tendons are exposed. The authors make a point of making sure the superior peroneal retinaculum is raised off the posterior fibula as a complete flap of tissue to help facilitate the reattachment with closure. At this point there should be good visualization of the very distal aspect of the fibula. The anterior talofibular ligament (ATFL) and calcaneofibular ligament (CFL) origin off the fibula may be difficult to identify with revision surgery because of the scarring and tissue attenuation. The ATFL and CFL are removed off the tip of the fibula as a complete flap of tissue avoiding damage to the peroneal tendons posteriorly.

The lateral aspect of the talus at the junction of the neck and body is visualized with minimal dissection. A soft tissue tunnel must be created for the graft between the peroneal tendons and the lateral wall of the calcaneus. This is accomplished by taking a key elevator or freer elevator to gently reflect the soft tissue (**Fig. 5**). The tunnel is normally about 1.0 to 1.5 cm in length. The lateral wall of the calcaneus is then exposed to identify the insertion location of the osseous tunnel for the graft. The peroneal tendons need to be retracted anterior to help with the exposure.

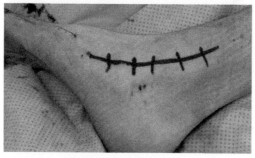

Fig. 4. Incisional approach for allograft reconstruction.

There are many choices of allografts for recreation of the ATFL and CFL. The authors prefer to use a peroneus longus allograft. The reasons for this is the graft is readily available, has enough length, and it gives the surgeon the option of either a round end or a flat end (**Fig. 6**). The graft is thawed in warm sterile saline for approximately 10 minutes before use. The authors have not found the need to "prestretch" the graft before insertion. Once the graft is thawed, the graft is then cut at the junction of the flat and the circular end to separate the two. The circular side is the one that is used most of the time.

An osseous tunnel is created from the tip of the lateral malleolus oriented proximally and either anteriorly or posteriorly so that the length of the tunnel is approximately 2.0 cm (**Fig. 7**). A 6-mm diameter tunnel is the most commonly used diameter. We have found that anything greater than this diameter runs the risk of breaking through the cortex of the fibula with insertion of the graft and biotenodesis screw. The graft is inserted into the fibular osseous tunnel and secured in place with a biotenodesis screw (**Fig. 8**). The graft is now carefully split into an anterior and posterior portion using a sharp #15 blade. A malleable retractor is used for a cutting surface and a hemostat is placed at the distal end of the graft to help keep tension on it. As the graft is cut from distal to proximal, be careful to keep the anterior and posterior halves as equal as possible. The splitting of the graft is stopped approximately 3 mm distal to the insertion of the graft into the fibula (**Fig. 9**).

Osseous tunnels are then placed into the calcaneus and talus for the posterior and anterior arms of the graft, respectively (**Fig. 10**). The location for the osseous tunnel of the talus is located at the junction of the body and neck of the talus. The ideal location for the tunnel is the center of the talus from superior to inferior. This is normally a 6-mm diameter tunnel. The location of the osseous tunnel within the calcaneus is directed 8mm inferior from the center of the posterior facet of the subtalar joint running in a lateral to medial direction (**Fig. 11**). The tunnel is oriented slight inferior. A 7-mm osseous tunnel is normally used, which allows for graft to be passed with ease.

Both arms of the grafts need to be shortened in order for proper tensioning of the ligament reconstruction. The surgeon must be careful not to overshorten the grafts. The most difficult graft to insert is the graft into the calcaneus, so the authors recommend starting with the CFL first. The posterior arm of the graft is passed under the peroneal tendons against the lateral wall of the calcaneus (**Fig. 12**). The graft is then placed into the calcaneus from lateral to medial. With the graft properly tensioned and the ankle joint held in a slightly exerted position, the graft is secured in place with a 7-mm biotenodesis screw (**Fig. 13**).

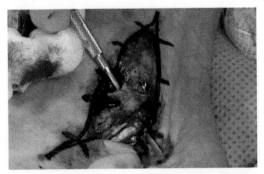

Fig. 5. Soft tissue tunnel inferior to the peroneal tendons for the allograft.

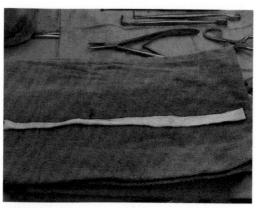

Fig. 6. Peroneal longus allograft.

The anterior arm is then placed into the osseous tunnel within the talus. The talus is positioned in a neutral position, the graft is tensioned, and secured in place with a 6 mm biotenodesis screw. With both grafts properly tensioned, the foot should maintain a neutral position when on the operating room table without any hands holding it in place (**Fig. 14**).

The incision is irrigated, and layered closure is performed. Closure involves relocation of the peroneal tendons and reattachment of the superior peroneal retinaculum. The soft tissue of the ATFL and CFL is also advanced over the graft and sutured in place using a 2–0 nonabsorbable suture. After skin closure, the foot and leg are placed in a postoperative sprint with the foot and ankle in neutral position.

Postoperative recovery is normally 2 weeks nonweightbearing in a splint followed by 2 weeks in a weightbearing cast as tolerated. At 4 weeks postoperative, the patient is advanced into a weightbearing boot. The boot is removed when sitting or sleeping but an ankle brace is applied to avoid excessive inversion and eversion. The patient can start to wean out of the boot using the ankle brace at 6 weeks postoperative. Physical therapy is typically started to assist the patient with slowly advancing activities and weaning out of the brace with walking. It is recommended that an ankle brace is

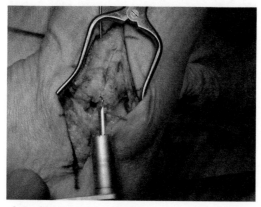

Fig. 7. Orientation of the fibula osseous tunnel.

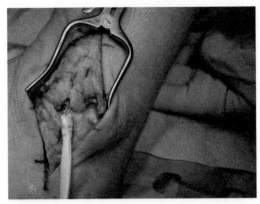

Fig. 8. Allograft insertion into the fibula.

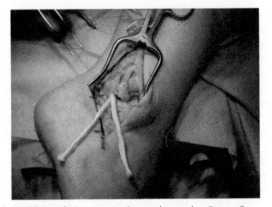

Fig. 9. Splitting of the allograft into posterior and anterior "arms."

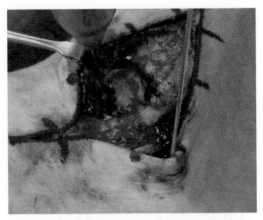

Fig. 10. Creation of the osseous tunnel into the calcaneus and talus.

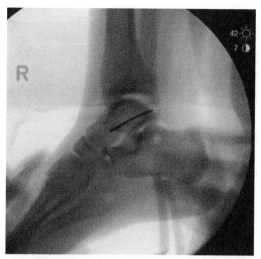

Fig. 11. Radiographic location of the osseous tunnels into the talus and calcaneus.

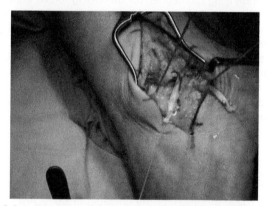

Fig. 12. Position of the allograft under the peroneal tendon sheath.

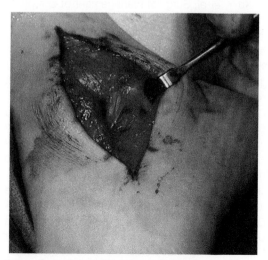

Fig. 13. Insertion of the allograft into the talus and calcaneus.

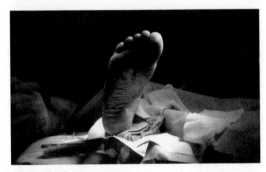

Fig. 14. Postoperative positioning.

used with sports that have a higher risk of inversion injuries, such as volleyball or basketball. Normally recovery takes approximately 4 to 6 months.

KEY SURGICAL POINTS

- Address any underlying biomechanical deforming forces either before the revision lateral ankle reconstruction or at the same time of the procedure.
- Be cautious not to shorten the allograft too much especially with the portion being inserted to the calcaneus.
- The allograft should insert easily into the osseous tunnels. It is better to have too large of a diameter osseous tunnel versus having to try and "stuff" the graft in a tunnel that is too small.
- Once the graft is inserted and tensioned, the ankle should stay in a neutral position on its own on the operating room table.

REFERENCES

1. Waterman BR, Owens BD, Davey S, et al. The epidemiology of ankle sprains in the United States. J Bone Joint Surg Am 2010;92(13):2279–84.
2. Colville MR. Surgical treatment of the unstable ankle. J Am Acad Orthop Surg 1998;6(6):368–77.
3. Cao Y, Hong Y, Xu Y, et al. Surgical management of chronic lateral ankle instability: a meta-analysis. J Orthop Surg Res 2018;13(1):159.
4. So E, Preston N, Holmes T. Intermediate- to long-term longevity and incidence of revision of the modified Brostrom-Gould procedure for lateral ankle ligament repair: a systematic review. J Foot Ankle Surg 2017;56(5):1076–80.
5. Bell SJ, Mologne TS, Sitler DF, et al. Twenty-six-year results after Brostrom procedure for chronic lateral ankle instability. Am J Sports Med 2006;34(6):975–8.
6. Brodsky AR, O'Malley MJ, Bohne WH, et al. An analysis of outcome measures following the Brostrom-Gould procedure for chronic lateral ankle instability. Foot Ankle Int 2005;26(10):816–9.
7. Hamilton WG, Thompson FM, Snow SW. The modified Brostrom procedure for lateral ankle instability. Foot Ankle 1993;14(1):1–7.
8. Karlsson J, Bergsten T, Lansinger O, et al. Reconstruction of the lateral ligaments of the ankle for chronic lateral instability. J Bone Joint Surg Am 1988;70(4):581–8.
9. Krips R, van Dijk CN, Halasi PT, et al. Long-term outcome of anatomical reconstruction versus tenodesis for the treatment of chronic anterolateral instability of the ankle joint: a multicenter study. Foot Ankle Int 2001;22(5):415–21.

10. Lee KT, Park YU, Kim JS, et al. Long-term results after modified Brostrom procedure without calcaneofibular ligament reconstruction. Foot Ankle Int 2011;32(2): 153–7.
11. Nielsen RH, Couppe C, Jensen JK, et al. Low tendon stiffness and abnormal ultrastructure distinguish classic Ehlers-Danlos syndrome from benign joint hypermobility syndrome in patients. FASEB J 2014;28(11):4668–76.
12. Park KH, Lee JW, Suh JW, et al. Generalized ligamentous laxity is an independent predictor of poor outcomes after the modified Brostrom procedure for chronic lateral ankle instability. Am J Sports Med 2016;44(11):2975–83.
13. Sammarco VJ. Complications of lateral ankle ligament reconstruction. Clin Orthop Relat Res 2001;391:123–32.
14. Messer TM, Cummins CA, Ahn J, et al. Outcome of the modified Brostrom procedure for chronic lateral ankle instability using suture anchors. Foot Ankle Int 2000;21(12):996–1003.
15. Petrera M, Dwyer T, Theodoropoulos JS, et al. Short- to medium-term outcomes after a modified Brostrom repair for lateral ankle instability with immediate postoperative weightbearing. Am J Sports Med 2014;42(7):1542–8.
16. Beighton P, Solomon L, Soskolne CL. Articular mobility in an African population. Ann Rheum Dis 1973;32(5):413–8.
17. DIGiovanni BF, Fraga CJ, Cohen BE, et al. Associated injuries found in chronic lateral ankle instability. Foot Ankle Int 2000;21(10):809–15.
18. Krause FG, Wing KJ, Younger AS. Neuromuscular issues in cavovarus foot. Foot Ankle Clin 2008;13(2):243–58, vi.
19. Larsen E, Angermann P. Association of ankle instability and foot deformity. Acta Orthop Scand 1990;61(2):136–9.
20. O'Neil JT, Guyton GP. Revision of surgical lateral ankle ligament stabilization. Foot Ankle Clin 2018;23(4):605–24.
21. Tyler TF, McHugh MP, Mirabella MR, et al. Risk factors for noncontact ankle sprains in high school football players: the role of previous ankle sprains and body mass index. Am J Sports Med 2006;34(3):471–5.
22. Xu HX, Lee KB. Modified Brostrom procedure for chronic lateral ankle instability in patients with generalized joint laxity. Am J Sports Med 2016;44(12):3152–7.
23. Gould N, Seligson D, Gassman J. Early and late repair of lateral ligament of the ankle. Foot Ankle 1980;1(2):84–9.
24. Kannus P, Renstrom P. Treatment for acute tears of the lateral ligaments of the ankle. Operation, cast, or early controlled mobilization. J Bone Joint Surg Am 1991;73(2):305–12.
25. Araoye I, Pinter Z, Lee S, et al. Revisiting the prevalence of associated copathologies in chronic lateral ankle instability: are there any predictors of outcome? Foot Ankle Spec 2019;12(4):311–5.
26. Okuda R, Kinoshita M, Morikawa J, et al. Arthroscopic findings in chronic lateral ankle instability: do focal chondral lesions influence the results of ligament reconstruction? Am J Sports Med 2005;33(1):35–42.
27. Choi WJ, Lee JW, Han SH, et al. Chronic lateral ankle instability: the effect of intraarticular lesions on clinical outcome. Am J Sports Med 2008;36(11):2167–72.
28. Diniz P, Pacheco J, Flora M, et al. Clinical applications of allografts in foot and ankle surgery. Knee Surg Sports Traumatol Arthrosc 2019;27(6):1847–72.
29. Li H, Song Y, Li H, et al. Outcomes after anatomic lateral ankle ligament reconstruction using allograft tendon for chronic ankle instability: a systematic review and meta-analysis. J Foot Ankle Surg 2020;59(1):117–24.

Revision of the Malaligned Ankle Arthrodesis

Christopher L. Reeves, DPM[a],*, Amber M. Shane, DPM[b], Hannah Sahli, DPM[c,1], Cody Togher, DPM[c,1]

KEYWORDS

- Malunion • Ankle arthrodesis • Revision • Malaligned fusion

KEY POINTS

- Understanding each component of the malaligned deformity is crucial to proper preoperative planning.
- Ideal position for ankle fusion is 0° to 5° of hindfoot valgus, neutral position in the sagittal plane, and 5° to 10° of external rotation as well as 1 cm of posterior talar displacement from the long axis of the tibia.
- Revision of the malaligned ankle fusion can be performed through closing wedge osteotomy, opening wedge osteotomy, focal dome osteotomy, external fixation, or total ankle arthroplasty.

INTRODUCTION

The maligned ankle arthrodesis is a rigid deformity that warrants considerable preparation when attempting revisional surgical correction. It is one of the leading causes of chronic postoperative pain after primary ankle arthrodesis and generates additional stress to adjacent joints, expediting their arthritic processes[1–8] (**Fig. 1**). These deformities often are extremely difficult to brace or treat with conservative methods, and surgical intervention often is utilized for definitive treatment. Surgical correction should be both symptom driven and deformity driven, and recent outcomes have shown results similar to those of primary procedures.[9–11] Due to the complex nature of this deformity, it may require multiple or staged procedures for adequate correction as well as correction of residual limb length discrepancy. The performing surgeon should

[a] Advent Health East Orlando Podiatric Surgery Residency, Orlando Foot and Ankle Clinic-Upperline Health, 2111 Glenwood Drive Suite 104, Winter Park, FL 32792, USA; [b] Department of Podiatric Surgery Advent Health System, Advent Health East Orlando Podiatric Surgery Residency, Orlando Foot and Ankle Clinic- Upperline Health, 250 North Alafaya Trail Suite 115, Orlando, FL 32828, USA; [c] Department of Podiatric Surgery AdventHealth System, Orlando, FL, USA
[1] Present address: 2111 Glenwood Drive Suite 104, Winter Park, FL 32792.
* Corresponding author.
E-mail address: Docreeves1@yahoo.com

Clin Podiatr Med Surg 37 (2020) 475–487
https://doi.org/10.1016/j.cpm.2020.03.003
0891-8422/20/© 2020 Elsevier Inc. All rights reserved.

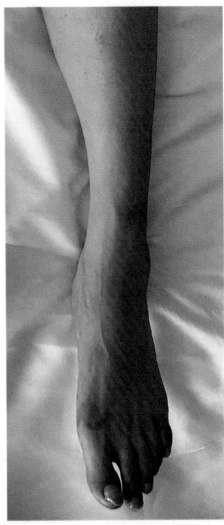

Fig. 1. Clinical view of a patient with a plantarflexed arthrodesis with severe atrophic changes.

also be aware of neglected deformity above or below the fusion mass, with accurate preoperative localization of the center of rotation of angulation (CORA) assisting in surgical correction.

Historically, reoperation rates for revisional ankle arthrodesis surgeries have been high, ranging between 50% and 70%.[12,13] In more recent literature, these procedures have shown good to excellent results, with outcomes similar to primary procedures with regard to union rates, patient satisfaction, and postoperative complications.[9–11] Limb length discrepancies commonly are reported and can be prevented during revisional procedures with the use of bone grafting or distraction osteogenesis techniques. With severe mispositioning, soft tissue procedures also should be considered to prevent additional postoperative complications and assist with surgical correction of the deformity.

Malalignment of the ankle joint during primary arthrodesis can be due to several factors. Neglection of the deforming soft tissue structures can cause undesirable forces across the fusion mass during the postoperative phases of bone healing, subsequently increasing the risk for pseudarthroses, hardware failure, and malalignment.[9,11] It is important to take these structures into account preoperatively because general anesthesia can cause intraoperative relaxation of musculotendinous structures, masking their potential effects on postoperative alignment. Asymmetric preparation of joint surfaces and failure to adequately resect osteonecrotic bone also can cause unfavorable positioning postoperatively.[9,14–17] In patients who undergo primary ankle arthrodesis for treatment of posttraumatic arthritis, symmetric resection of all nonviable bone is key to preventing residual deformities. Necrotic bone has low healing potential, and failure to adequately resect bone can lead to poor apposition of the fusion mass and subsequent malalignment or nonunion.[14–17] Charcot neuroarthropathy also has been shown related to nonunion and deformity after primary ankle arthrodesis in neuropathic patients. In this population, revisional surgery can be performed when limb salvage is appropriate.

A multitude of procedures have been described for correction of the malaligned ankle arthrodesis. Techniques ranging from opening wedge osteotomies to utilization of realignment external fixation devices all have been described in the literature. This article reviews proper positioning of ankle arthrodesis and issues associated with planar deformities after fusion of the talocrural joint. Additionally, surgical options for revision of the malaligned ankle arthrodesis are discussed and recent findings in the literature associated with these techniques analyze. With a good knowledge base and the proper attention to detail, revisional surgery for the malaligned ankle arthrodesis can have excellent outcomes when performed by a well-trained surgeon.

CORRECT POSITIONING

Proper positioning for ankle joint arthrodesis has been researched extensively in the literature.[9,18–22] Collectively, these studies have agreed that 0° to 5° of hindfoot valgus, neutral positioning of the ankle in the sagittal plane, and 5° to 10° of external rotation is the desired position for a successful ankle fusion. Several investigators also have studied the advantages of posterior talar displacement 1 cm relative to the long axis of the tibia. They have found this alignment optimizes the lever arm of the lower extremity by shortening the unit as a whole and is beneficial for decreasing energy expenditure during the swing phase of gait[18–22] (Fig. 2).

Total energy expense is decreased, with the ankle fused with the foot in this alignment. This positioning contributes to both radiographic and clinical outcomes as well as long-term patient satisfaction.[18–22] Waters and colleagues[22] found gait efficiency to be 90% with ankle joint arthrodesis in this position. Available compensation for other joints is highest in this alignment, and it has proved to provide less strain on ipsilateral knee joints.[21] Furthermore, stride length and gait velocity were found less affected when this position is achieved. Although historically the hypothetical norms for ankle positioning has been up for debate, the current accepted positioning has been in place for the past 40 years.[21]

EFFECTS OF MALALIGNED ANKLE ARTHRODESIS

The presence of planar deformities after ankle joint arthrodesis can be damning to postoperative outcomes. Asymmetric loading of the lower extremity combined with excessive motion to adjacent joints predisposes patients to the development of pressure wounds, stress risers and fractures, hardware failure, osteoarthritis, and

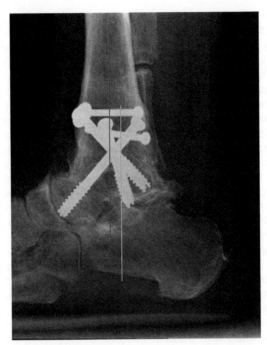

Fig. 2. Radiograph of an ankle arthrodesis with varus malalignment.

ultimately nonunion with or without pseudarthrosis of the fusion site. These complications provide a challenge to treat conservatively due to the rigidity of the deformity and lack of available compensatory motion to the ipsilateral knee and small joints of the foot. In preparation for surgical revision, the performing surgeon should first be familiar with the common complications associated with deformities in each of the cardinal planes as well as how to properly identify of the CORA of the deformity being corrected.

Frontal Plane Deformities

Frontal plane positioning of the ankle and hindfoot is essential for postoperative outcomes after arthrodesis of the talocrural joint. Blackwood and colleagues and later Desilva and Gill further explained Elftman's original theory which suggests that hindfoot positioning dictates both forefoot position as well as overall motion available to the midtarsal joints.[23–25] When the hindfoot is supinated, the axes of motion of the midtarsal joints become more parallel, decreasing available range of motion and ability of adjacent joints to compensate. Elftman also believed that the maximally pronated position of the midtarsal joint is parallel to that of the subtalar joint, meaning that if the ankle and subtalar joint are in varus alignment, the maximally pronated position of the forefoot will remain in this position as well. Although there is conflicting evidence supporting this theory,[26–28] it may help explain why any degree of varus alignment after ankle joint arthrodesis typically is considered unfavorable and can be more challenging to treat conservatively.

Varus deformities of the ankle joint are often associated with an increased incidence of nonunion (see **Fig. 2**). A study in 2015 by Chalayon and colleagues[29] found a 2-fold increase in the risk of nonunion after ankle joint arthrodesis with a preoperative varus alignment. Patients who have undergone ankle joint arthrodesis with a residual varus deformity frequently present with complaints related to overloading of the lateral column. Fifth metatarsal stress fractures, cuboid subluxation, and pressure wounds over the lateral malleolus or styloid process of the fifth metatarsal are recurring complications in this population. Lateral ankle pain can occur secondary to peroneal spasm and overuse in attempt to guard painful arthritic motion at the subtalar joint, while also hyperpronating the medial column in an attempt to distribute the ground reactive forces equally throughout the foot.

A mild valgus position of the ankle joint often is recommended during arthrodesis because it allows for more shock absorption and compensatory motion to the midfoot. Midfoot motion is of special importance after ankle joint arthrodesis because a majority of compensatory pedal dorsiflexions occur here after ankle joint arthrodesis. Valgus positioning greater than 5° can lead to postoperative medial knee pain, progression of genu valgum, pes planus deformities, and arthritis to the midfoot secondary to excessive motion.[1-7]

Sagittal Plane-specific Complications

Although less challenging to treat via conservative methods, sagittal plane deformities after ankle joint arthrodesis can be equally problematic if left unaddressed. Patients with postoperative equinus deformities typically develop painful hyperkeratosis plantar to the metatarsal heads and experience metatarsalgia secondary to overloading of the forefoot (**Fig. 3**). Stress fractures of the second metatarsal are not uncommon, and progression of midtarsal joint osteoarthritis and pes planus typically are seen. Conversely, patients who have dorsiflexory deformities after ankle joint arthrodesis tend to have complaints of heel pain with the possibility for calcaneal stress fractures from consistent overloading and fat pad atrophy of the hindfoot[30] (**Fig. 4**).

Transverse Plane-specific Complications

Deformities in the transverse plane are less symptomatic than those in the other 2 cardinal planes. As expected, these deformities frequently develop complaints secondary to axial compensation of the knee and hip, causing varying levels of pain and arthritis in these areas. Treatment of symptoms usually is successful in most cases, with revisional surgical correction of transverse plane deformities typically occurring only when the deformity is multiplanar.

Translational deformities should also be considered when attempting revisional surgical correction of a malaligned ankle arthrodesis. One centimeter of posterior displacement of the talus beneath the tibia is advantageous for gait efficiency after ankle joint arthrodesis but not essential to overall outcomes or development of complications.[9,18-22] Imsdahl and colleagues in 2019 performed cadaveric gait simulations that showed anteroposterior displacement greater than 6 mm can cause significant increases in aberrant joint loading, ultimately contributing to poor outcomes and increased incidence of adjacent joint arthritis.[31]

Identification of the Center of Rotation of Angulation

A systematic approach to the surgical revision of the malaligned ankle arthrodesis should include accurate identification of the apex of the deformity, or CORA. Advanced imaging, including computerized tomography, is imperative in the guidance of surgical revision as well as in how to interpret the information necessary for surgical planning. Using the techniques described by Paley,[32] the surgeon can pinpoint the intersection of the proximal and distal mechanical axes of the combined tibiotalar unit to properly assess the CORA; consequently, evaluation of the angle between these 2 axes assists in quantifying the degree of deformity[32,33] (**Fig. 5**). In a successful

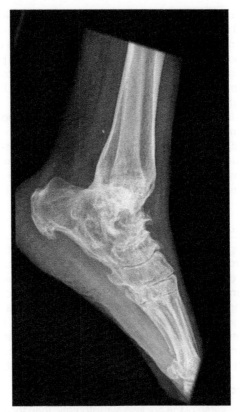

Fig. 3. Radiographic view of a plantarflexed ankle arthrodesis.

arthrodesis, where deformity is present, surgical correction is directed at the location of CORA. This differs from cases of nonunion present and needs to be addressed. In these instances, translation often is required in addition to correction of angular and rotational components to successfully realign the lower extremity. Although CORA

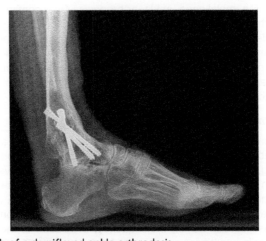

Fig. 4. Radiograph of a dorsiflexed ankle arthrodesis.

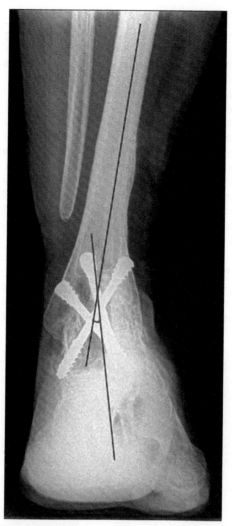

Fig. 5. Depicts measurement of CORA.

may be the ideal location for correction, the surgeon must consider the quality of soft tissue envelope, healing potential of osteotomized bone, location of remaining internal fixation, and the ability to place new rigid fixation.

REVISIONAL SURGICAL OPTIONS

Once full understanding of the patient-specific deformity is achieved, correction then requires 3 decisions: the location of the osteotomy, the type of osteotomy, and the method of stabilization. The location of the osteotomy must be based on the site of deformity and biological factors of the patient. Closing and opening wedge osteotomies, focal dome osteotomies, callus distraction, and total ankle replacement all are within the surgeon's armamentarium for revision of a malaligned ankle.

Closing Wedge Osteotomy

Closing wedge osteotomy is the most common method for angular correction. This osteotomy is able to correct directly at the site of deformity while resulting in viable bone on bone contact. This osteotomy can be made with precise cuts and allow for autograft bone if any other procedures are being performed.[30,34] A disadvantage to this approach includes functionally lengthening the surrounding tendinous structures associated to changes in limb length. To perform a closing wedge osteotomy of the tibia, surgeons should focus their attention to concave side of the intersections between the proximal and distal mechanical axes. This is important because the concavity of the deformity serves as the rotational point of correction. Once the rotational axis has been identified, a line then is drawn perpendicular to both the mechanical axes (as measured on both anteroposterior and lateral radiographs). These perpendicular lines create the hypothetical wedge of bone to be removed for deformity correction (**Fig. 6**). The length lost in the limb is equal to one-half the height of the wedge's base.[34] Once the wedge is removed, the bone segments are brought together and fixated with surgeon's preference of internal or external fixation.

Opening Wedge Osteotomy

In contrast to closing wedge, opening wedge osteotomy provides another option. The advantage of an opening wedge osteotomy is the ability to regain length and restore the anatomic and functional relationships between musculotendinous structures. In

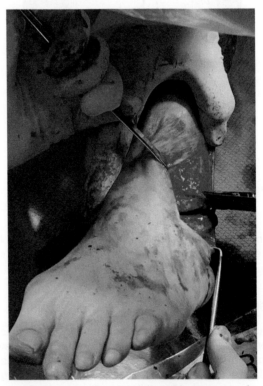

Fig. 6. Closing wedge osteotomy performed through fusion mass of a plantarflexed malunion. The wedge was created anteriorly with a posterior hinge.

2003, Probe[34] demonstrated that the length gained during opening wedge osteotomies is equal to one-half the height of the distracted triangular base. Disadvantages to this approach include strain on surrounding neurovascular structures and high risk of nonunion owing to the need of a large allograft wedge. An opening wedge osteotomy should be discouraged in patients who have diabetes or rheumatoid arthritis or who are current smokers.[35] To perform an opening wedge osteotomy for varus deformity, the incision is placed on the medial side of the tibia (either at CORA or 5 cm proximal to the ankle joint). At this level, a transverse osteotomy is performed perpendicular to the long axis of the tibia. Next, a lamina spreader is placed and gently distracted, allowing the osteotomy to correct the deformity. The magnitude of distraction is based on preoperative measurements and intraoperative fluoroscopy. The resulting gap then is filled with an allograft bone wedge. An asymmetric graft also may be placed to achieve multiplanar correction. Lastly, the site is spanned with a plate for rigid internal fixation.[35]

Focal Dome Osteotomy

Focal dome osteotomies provide the ability to dial in correction about a central point of rotation. Dome osteotomies traditionally are placed in metaphyseal area utilizing the bone healing potential of the cancellous bone in this region. Advantages specific to focal dome osteotomies include lack of thermal necrosis, minimal periosteal dissection, and inherent stability due to excellent bone-to-bone contact. This technique also minimizes loss in tibial length.[33] To perform this osteotomy, a half-pin is placed as close to CORA as possible in metaphyseal bone, perpendicular to the long axis of the tibia. For varus/valgus deformities, the pin is placed from anterior to posterior; however, with sagittal plane deformities the pin is placed from medial to lateral.

When treating a malaligned ankle fusion, the CORA may be at the ankle joint. If this is the case, the pin should be placed just proximal to the joint line. Next, a radial lever arm guide is applied to the half pin and used as a template. The guide must be positioned to ensure the osteotomy exits both cortices. Multiple percutaneous drill holes are then placed along the guide through small skin incisions. The drill holes begin to form a dome-like appearance (**Fig. 7**); an osteotome then is used to complete the osteotomy (**Fig. 8**). Next, the foot and ankle distal to the osteotomy are manipulated to rotate about the dome correcting the deformity.[33] Once correction is achieved using careful intraoperative fluoroscopy, rigid internal fixation is applied.

External Fixation

External fixation often is utilized in revision of malaligned ankle arthrodesis. It may be warranted for primary fixation or augmentation internal fixation or as a means of correction through callus distraction techniques. In cases of extreme or multiplanar deformity or cases of significant limb shortening present, gradual correction should be considered.[30] When attempting correction through callus distraction, a multilevel external fixator with hinges allows for custom correction. This method often is utilized in attempt to restore anatomic length and alignment in complex deformities. The hinges of this construct serve as a point of rotational correction by creating a trapezoidal opening wedge.[30] After placement of the external ring fixator with telescoping struts, a computer-based program can be used to map out rate of distraction to achieve desired correction. Although computer-based programming makes this complex process easier, it still should be reserved for complex deformities in patients who can tolerate external fixation for an extended period of time.

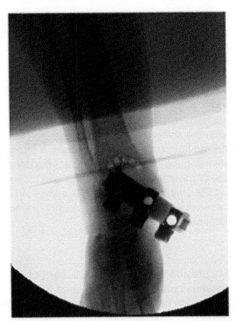

Fig. 7. Intraoperative radiographic view of a focal dome osteotomy. The pin was placed centrally within the tibia and the guide positioned to ensure drill holes exit the tibial cortices. A drill then was used to create a dome.

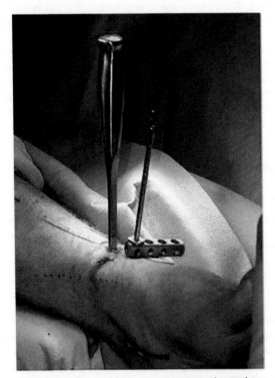

Fig. 8. Through percutaneous skin incisions an osteotome is used to complete the focal dome osteotomy.

Total Ankle Replacement

Revision of the malaligned ankle arthrodesis via conversion to total ankle arthroplasty (TAA) is a topic that has consistently gained momentum since the beginning of the millennium. Although earlier studies had reported high incidence of medial malleolar fracture and high rate of additional procedures after initial conversion, they have continued to show improved results over time.[7,10,36] In 2016, Huntington and colleagues[37] published a small case series of 5 patients who underwent conversion of ankle arthrodesis to TAA, with 80% of patients having satisfactory outcomes. The next year, Preis and colleagues[38] also published a study reviewing 20 patients who underwent the same procedure in treatment of ankle arthrodesis nonunion or malunion. Their research reported not only lower incidence of periprosthetic fractures but also increased procedural success compared with more recent studies and decreased rate or return of surgery after conversion to TAA.[38] Preis and colleagues[39] followed this study up with another in 2019, this time investigating TAA conversion from tibiotalocalcaneal arthrodesis. Again they demonstrated favorable results, further suggesting its efficacy as a surgical treatment option.[39] These studies not only support conversion to TAA but also reinforce its place as a successful and viable option in the surgical revision of a malaligned ankle arthrodesis.

When performing TAA in the treatment of a malaligned ankle arthrodesis, there are several important tips and pearls to keep in mind. Arguably, the most important of these is the surgeon's ability to accurately perform the arthrodesis takedown osteotomy at the level of the previous joint line. This vital step not only helps to guide placement of the implant and assist in the correction of residual deformity but also assists in preservation of limb length and prevention of malleolar fractures. Computerized tomography of both the affected limb and contralateral limb is recommended for accurate triangulation of the previous joint line. Additionally, prophylactic pinning of the malleoli often is implemented intraoperatively to prevent periprosthetic or malleolar fracturing. Several different techniques have been described in the literature for conversion of malaligned ankle arthrodesis into TAA.[8,40,41] Utilization of some of these techniques may assist good long-term results when performed by a skilled surgeon.

SUMMARY

A malaligned ankle fusion is a rigid deformity that can be both physically and emotionally debilitating to the patient. Correct positioning is crucial to both short-term and long-term outcomes. Deformity may present itself in the coronal, sagittal, or transverse plane or a combination of the cardinal planes. The key to success in revising a malaligned ankle fusion comes from thorough understanding of this rigid and complex deformity, including identification of CORA. Surgeons then can assess the patient as a whole by managing expectations, goals, soft tissue envelope, and biologic healing ability to choose the best route of revision. Utilization of these principles gives the surgeon a multitude of options in the revision of malaligned ankle arthrodesis. Closing wedge osteotomies, opening wedge osteotomies, focal dome osteotomies, callus distraction, or total ankle replacement can be performed. Extensive preoperative planning is required for complete resolution of this complex deformity but when done appropriately can lead to an ambulating, satisfied patient.

DISCLOSURE

The doctors have nothing to disclose.

REFERENCES

1. Sturnick DR, Demetracopoulos CA, Ellis SJ, et al. Adjacent joint kinematics after ankle arthrodesis during cadaveric gait simulation. Foot Ankle Int 2017;38(11): 1249–59.
2. Bruening DA, Cooney TE, Ray MS, et al. Multisegment foot kinematic and kinetic compensations in level and uphill walking following tibiotalar arthrodesis. Foot Ankle Int 2016;37(10):1119–29.
3. Beyaert C, Sirveaux F, Paysant J, et al. The effect of tibio-talar arthrodesis on foot kinematics and ground reaction force progression during walking. Gait Posture 2004;20(1):84–91.
4. Valderrabano V, Hintermann B, Nigg BM, et al. Kinematic changes after fusion and total replacement of the ankle part 1: range of motion. Foot Ankle Int 2003; 24(12):881–7.
5. Valderrabano V, Hintermann B, Nigg BM, et al. Kinematic changes after fusion and total replacement of the ankle part 2: movement transfer. Foot Ankle Int 2003;24(12):888–96.
6. Wayne JS, Lawhorn KW, Davis KE, et al. The effect of tibiotalar fixation on foot biomechanics. Foot Ankle Int 1997;18(12):792–7.
7. Greisberg J, Assal M, Flueckiger G, et al. Takedown of ankle fusion and conversion to total ankle replacement. Clin Orthop Relat Res 2004;424:80–8.
8. Devries JG, Hyer CF, Berlet GC. Ankle Arthrodesis and Malunion Takedown to Total Ankle Replacement. Primary and Revision Total Ankle Replacement. 2015:395–405. https://doi.org/10.1007/978-3-319-24415-0_34.
9. Midis N, Conti SF. Revision ankle arthrodesis. Foot Ankle Int 2002;23(3):243–7.
10. Barg A, Hintermann B. Takedown of painful ankle fusion and total ankle replacement using a 3-component ankle prosthesis. Tech Foot Ankle Surg 2010;9(4): 190–8.
11. O'Connor KM, Johnson JE, Mccormick JJ, et al. Clinical and operative factors related to successful revision arthrodesis in the foot and ankle. Foot Ankle Int 2016;37(8):809–15.
12. Morgan CD, Henke JA, Bailey RW, et al. Long-term results of tibiotalar arthrodesis. J Bone Joint Surg Am 1985;67(4):546–50.
13. Lance EM, Paval A, Fries I, et al. Arthrodesis of the ankle joint. Clin Orthop Relat Res 1979;(142):146–58.
14. Dimitriou R, Jones E, Mcgonagle D, et al. Bone regeneration: current concepts and future directions. BMC Med 2011;9(1). https://doi.org/10.1186/1741-7015-9-66.
15. Kodama N, Takemura Y, Shioji S, et al. Arthrodesis of the ankle using an anterior sliding tibial graft for osteoarthritis secondary to osteonecrosis of the talus. Bone Joint J 2016;98-B(3):359–64.
16. Lachman JR, Adams SB. Tibiotalocalcaneal arthrodesis for severe talar avascular necrosis. Foot Ankle Clin 2019;24(1):143–61.
17. Bergeyk AV, Stotler W, Beals T, et al. Functional outcome after modified blair tibiotalar arthrodesis for talar osteonecrosis. Foot Ankle Int 2003;24(10):765–70.
18. Hefti FL, Baumann JRU, Morscher EW. Ankle joint fusion? Determination of optimal position by gait analysis. Arch Orthop Trauma Surg 1980;96(3):187–95.
19. Scranton PE, Fu FH, Brown TD. Ankle arthrodesis. Clin Orthop Relat Res 1980;(151). https://doi.org/10.1097/00003086-198009000-00034.
20. Mazur JM, Schwartz E, Simon SR. Ankle arthrodesis. Long-term follow-up with gait analysis. J Bone Joint Surg Am 1979;61(7):964–75.

21. Buck P, Morrey BF, Chao EY. The optimum position of arthrodesis of the ankle. A gait study of the knee and ankle. J Bone Joint Surg Am 1987;69(7):1052–62.
22. Waters RL, Barnes G, Husserl T, et al. Comparable energy expenditure after arthrodesis of the hip and ankle. J Bone Joint Surg Am 1988;70(7):1032–7.
23. Desilva JM, Gill SV. Brief communication: a midtarsal (midfoot) break in the human foot. Am J Phys Anthropol 2013;151(3):495–9.
24. Elftman H. The transverse tarsal joint and its control. Clin Orthop 1960;16:41–6.
25. Blackwood CB, Yuen TJ, Sangeorzan BJ, et al. The midtarsal joint locking mechanism. Foot Ankle Int 2005;26(12):1074–80.
26. Phan C-B, Shin G, Lee KM, et al. Skeletal kinematics of the midtarsal joint during walking: midtarsal joint locking revisited. J Biomech 2019;95:109287.
27. Nester CJ, Findlow A, Bowker P. Scientific approach to the axis of rotation at the midtarsal joint. J Am Podiatr Med Assoc 2001;91(2):68–73.
28. Okita N, Meyers SA, Challis JH, et al. Midtarsal joint locking: new perspectives on an old paradigm. J Orthop Res 2013;32(1):110–5.
29. Chalayon O, Wang B, Blankenhorn B, et al. Factors affecting the outcomes of uncomplicated primary open ankle arthrodesis. Foot Ankle Int 2015;36(10):1170–9.
30. Raikin SM, Rampuri V. An approach to the failed ankle arthrodesis. Foot Ankle Clin 2008;13(3):401–16.
31. Imsdahl SI, Stender CJ, Cook BK, et al. Anteroposterior translational malalignment of ankle arthrodesis alters foot biomechanics in cadaveric gait simulation. J Orthop Res 2019. https://doi.org/10.1002/jor.24464.
32. Paley D. Frontal Plane Mechanical and Anatomic Axis Planning. Principles of Deformity Correction. 2002:61–97. https://doi.org/10.1007/978-3-642-59373-4_4.
33. Mendicino RW, Catanzariti AR, Reeves CL. Percutaneous supramalleolar osteotomy for distal tibial (near articular) ankle deformities. J Am Podiatr Med Assoc 2005;95(1):72–84.
34. Probe RA. Correction of lower extremity angular malunion. Oper Tech Orthop 2003;13(2):120–9.
35. Benthien RA, Myerson MS. Supramalleolar osteotomy for ankle deformity and arthritis. Foot Ankle Clin 2004;9(3):475–87.
36. Hintermann B, Barg A, Knupp M, et al. Conversion of painful ankle arthrodesis to total ankle arthroplasty. J Bone Joint Surg Am 2009;91(4):850–8.
37. Huntington WP, Davis WH, Anderson R. Total ankle arthroplasty for the treatment of symptomatic nonunion following tibiotalar fusion. Foot Ankle Spec 2016;9(4):330–5.
38. Preis M, Bailey T, Marchand LS, et al. Can a three-component prosthesis be used for conversion of painful ankle arthrodesis to total ankle replacement? Clin Orthop Relat Res 2017;475(9):2283–94.
39. Preis M, Bailey T, Marchand LS, et al. Conversion of painful tibiotalocalcaneal arthrodesis to total ankle replacement using a 3-component mobile bearing prosthesis. Foot Ankle Surg 2019;25(3):286–93.
40. Hintermann B, Barg A, Knupp M, et al. Conversion of painful ankle arthrodesis to total ankle arthroplasty. surgical technique. J Bone Joint Surg Am 2010;92(Suppl 1):55–66.
41. Schuberth JM, Christensen JC, Seidenstricker C. Takedown of ankle arthrodesis with insufficient fibula: surgical technique and intermediate-term follow-up. J Foot Ankle Surg 2018;57(2):216–20.

Revision Surgery for Failed Total Ankle Replacement

Byron Hutchinson, DPM*, Mallory J. Schweitzer, DPM, MHA

KEYWORDS

- Circular fixation • Femoral head allograft • Custom trabecular metal cages
- Segmental bone defect • Total ankle replacement

KEY POINTS

- Total ankle explant involves some degree of bone loss and the segmental bone defect complicates reconstruction.
- Determination of aseptic versus infective loosening is paramount.
- Management of deformity and limb length discrepancy must be considered.

INTRODUCTION

In the past 10 years there has been a resurgence of interest in total ankle replacement (TAR) in select patients with end-stage ankle arthritis.[1] Survivorship for the most recent generation of ankle prostheses has improved, but failure rates remain higher than those seen in hip and knee replacements.[2–4] A number of total ankle replacement patients will require revisions at or within 10 years. Components have been designed to deal with some TAR revisions, but explanting the device may be the best option for certain patients. This article discusses the considerations for TAR explant and provides options available based on some specific guidelines developed by the lead author (B.H.).

AUTHORS' INDICATIONS FOR TOTAL ANKLE REPLACEMENT EXPLANT

There are several indications for TAR explant. The most common is aseptic loosening of the various components. Aseptic loosening can be managed with a TAR revision surgery but in some circumstances explant is a better option, especially in cases of considerable bone loss or a limb length discrepancy. If there is significant subsidence of the talus, the remaining bone may not be amenable to revision components and explant may be a more appropriate option. Patients who have significant osteoporosis or osteopenia that have been implanted may not be able to support revision components in a TAR and actually may do better with an explant. The author (B.H.) has seen

CHI Franciscan, 16233 Sylvester Road Southwest, Suite G-10, Burien, WA 98166, USA
* Corresponding author.
E-mail address: ByronHutchinson@CHIFranciscan.org

Clin Podiatr Med Surg 37 (2020) 489–504
https://doi.org/10.1016/j.cpm.2020.03.004
0891-8422/20/© 2020 Elsevier Inc. All rights reserved.

this in patients with inflammatory arthropathy. Periprosthetic infection also causes loosening and is another indication for TAR explant. Septic fusion with or without a lengthening has been shown to have good outcomes after implant infection. Significant deformity in the foot and/or tibia can compromise a TAR and the author (B.H.) has seen cases of this not addressed prior to the index surgery. This makes it more difficult to predict outcomes with revision of the TAR, and either a staged revision procedure addressing the deformity or an explant should be considered. Lastly, chronic pain after TAR does occur, even if the components are intact and there is relatively good motion. Gutter débridement, injections, and bracing can benefit some of these patients, but in some rare circumstances the author (B.H.) has found that explant is an appropriate option.

GENERAL SURGICAL CONSIDERATIONS

Many factors influence procedure selection when considering revision or explant after TAR failure. Deformity in both the foot and ankle must be addressed during the reconstruction. Patients also should be evaluated for any supramalleolar deformity that may not have been appreciated prior to the index procedure. There is a limb length discrepancy after explant due to bone loss and it has been well documented that discrepancies of greater than 10 mm can cause low back pain and hip pain.[5] The stability and alignment of the implant also must be considered. Certainly, if the components are stable, then exchange of the polyethylene insert may be all that is necessary. In cases of component failure, assessment of the integrity of the bone, structural malalignment, and loosening must be considered[6,7] (**Fig. 1**). When an implant appears loose on imaging or the alignment of the implant has shifted, it is critical to rule out infection as a cause of loosening. The discussion of proximal amputation is necessary in these cases, even if it is not imminent.

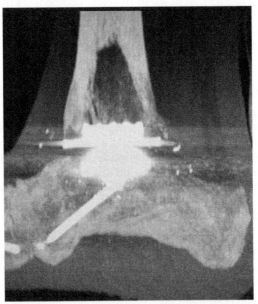

Fig. 1. Sagittal CT scan indicating stress shielding above the tibial component in a failed TAR.

SPECIFIC SURGICAL CONSIDERATIONS

In the face of implant failure, the decisions for the surgeon and patient can be challenging. Age of the patients and their health status must be considered. Some patients are not good candidates for multiple revision surgeries or may not tolerate multiple procedures. The condition of the soft tissue envelope also may limit the surgical options and preoperatively should be assessed thoroughly. In the author's (B.H.) experience, TAR explant in patients with rheumatoid arthritis is much more challenging than in patients who have posttraumatic arthritis or osteoarthritis in terms of revision and/or explant.[8,9]

Aseptic loosening occurs more often in TAR than in total hip and knee arthroplasty.[2] One of the contributing factors for aseptic loosening is motion at the bone-implant interface that affects bone ingrowth into the porous-surfaced implants.[10,11] It is the author's (B.H.) experience that there is little bony ingrowth on the components in a vast majority of the implants that are removed (**Fig. 2**).

Chronic periprosthetic infection also can contribute to loosening of the implant components, and infection needs to be ruled out in any cases of implant loosening. This is extremely important because infection limits the types of explant conversion techniques that are available. Both aseptic loosening and infection present with nonspecific progressive pain and the clinical situation can be very similar. Cases of subacute or chronic periprosthetic infections often do not present with local or systemic signs of infection. Previous records may be helpful in determining if there was an acute periprosthetic infection or a wound dehiscence present at the time of the index surgery, and this should increase suspicion that the implant is in fact infected.

Imaging studies and laboratory tests should be obtained to help differentiate between aseptic versus infective loosening but the definitive tests are periprosthetic tissue and bone samples for culture and biopsy. Identification of two positive periprosthetic cultures with phenotypically identical microorganisms is definitive along with bone biopsy changes indicating chronic osteomyelitis. In addition, serum interleukin-6 has 97% accuracy and 100% specificity in periprosthetic infections.[12] After explant, the components can be sonicated to determine if there are bacteria present.

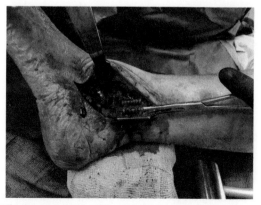

Fig. 2. Removal of tibial component with minimal osseous ingrowth.

TOTAL ANKLE REPLACEMENT EXPLANT WITH PERIPROSTHETIC INFECTION

When infection has been confirmed, the surgeon has 4 reconstructive options to consider. The antibiotic therapy generally is the same for all of these options and typically is parenteral for 6 weeks to 8 weeks with the appropriate antibiotics. The first option is explant with antibiotic spacer followed by reimplantation in 6 months to 12 months, when the infection has been eradicated. The second option is grafting using the Masquelet technique whereby the components are removed and there is maintenance of the segmental bone defect with an antibiotic spacer and circular fixator for 4 weeks. The spacer then is removed, maintaining the biologic membrane, and the segmental bone defect is packed with cancellous bone graft.[13] The third option is explant and primary septic fusion with or without tibial lengthening. This is accomplished by using circular fixation to simultaneously compress the fusion site and lengthen the tibia either proximally or distally, in cases of lengthening desired. This is discussed in greater detail later. The final option is a definitive amputation.

TOTAL ANKLE REPLACEMENT EXPLANT WITHOUT INFECTION

When explant is considered and infection has been ruled out, there are several options available to the foot and ankle surgeon. The critical decision to moving forward with a specific technique depends on the amount of bone loss at the time of the explant. It also is important to understand whether the bone loss involves both the tibia and talus or if it just the individual segments. Once this has been evaluated, the size of the segmental defect can be determined. This aids in deciding which explant technique is the most appropriate given the clinical situation.

Historically, utilization of a femoral head allograft in conjunction with plating or intramedullary (IM) nail fixation has been described.[14,15] Most of the literature has been operative techniques, case reports, or small series presentations. More recent publications have shown 50% failure rates using bulk allograft.[16,17] This has been the author's (B.H.) experience as well with large bulk allograft. Graft failure appears to be correlated to the size of the graft. Creep at the edges of the graft occurs and there is dissolution of the center of the graft, resulting in collapse (**Figs. 3** and **4**). Intercalary bone grafting can still be appropriate in some cases when the segmental bone defect is 2 cm or less.

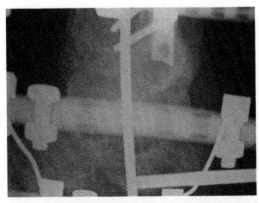

Fig. 3. Bulk femoral head allograft used in a TAR explant with circular fixation. Radiograph appears to show incorporation 4 months postoperatively and frame was removed.

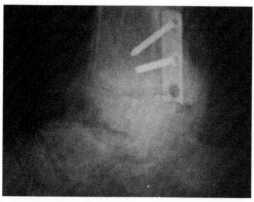

Fig. 4. Bulk femoral allograft dissolution at 6 months after circular frame removal.

Alternatives to bulk femoral head allograft have become popular in recent years with reasonable outcomes.[18–24] Newer implant options include custom trabecular metal cages and porous tantalum spacers. These devices are encouraging in many situations and can be combined with IM nails or plating systems for stability (**Fig. 5**). Many of these techniques are combined with various orthobiologics, autogenous bone graft, allogeneic bone graft, or a combination of these to facilitate osteoinduction, osteoconduction, and osteogenesis. There are few evidenced-based studies to support the use of any of these products in this setting. Given that these are revision cases and failure may require amputation, however, the author (B.H.) feels justified in using these orthobiologics in an attempt to enhance outcomes.

Circular external fixation may be useful or necessary in cases of TAR explant. Bifocal treatment with talocalcaneal (TC) fusion in conjunction with proximal or distal distraction osteogenisis has been described as a useful option in these difficult cases (**Figs. 6–10**).[25–28] This technique provides the advantages of predictable regenerate formation and consolidation of a primary fusion. Circular fixation also can be utilized with a compromised soft tissue envelope, which is common in these cases.[29] Often there is poor bone quality, and the stability provided by the external fixator and the

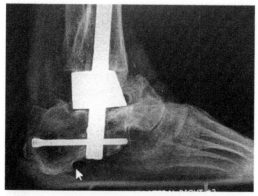

Fig. 5. Radiograph at 2 years postoperatively of TAR explant with tantalum spacer filled with autogenous bone graft and IM nail. Note the anterior fusion from grafting and no sign of failure of the spacer or nail.

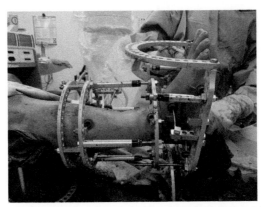

Fig. 6. Construct of circular external fixator for primary tibiocalcaneal fusion and simultaneous tibial distraction osteogenesis.

ability to dynamize the frame improves bony consolidation.[30,31] In addition, studies have shown that a corticotomy above a fusion site increases blood flow and aids in fusion.[32] Circular fixation also addresses the limb length inherent in these cases as well as any deformity that might be present. It also is the gold standard in the face of periprosthetic infection.

Utilization of an antibiotic spacer as a definitive option also can be considered in some patients who are low demand and may have comorbidities that preclude a major reconstruction. There is some support for this option and the author (B.H.) has found this the best option in a select number of patients.[33,34] In cases of the antibiotic spacer intended to be used as definitive treatment, the author (B.H.) fashions the spacer with short proximal and distal stems that are impacted into the tibia and talus or calcaneus to attempt to increase stability and limit movement of the spacer.

PROPOSED GUIDELINES FOR TOTAL ANKLE REPLACEMENT EXPLANT

The following guidelines for TAR explant have been developed by the author (B.H.) to provide some direction when considering surgery in these extremely complex cases

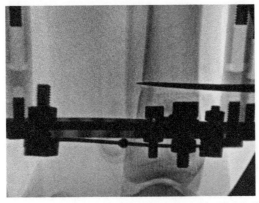

Fig. 7. Intraoperative fluoroscopic image of the placement of a distal tibial corticotomy for lengthening of the tibia.

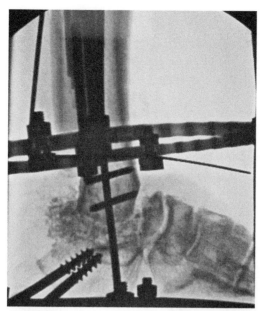

Fig. 8. Lateral fluoroscopic image of consolidated tibiocalcaneal fusion with foot plate removed to allow weight-bearing for dynamization of the tibial regenerate.

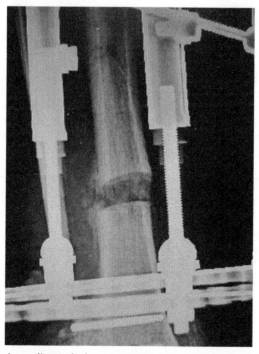

Fig. 9. Anteroposterior radiograph demonstrating consolidation of tibial regenerate while still in the frame.

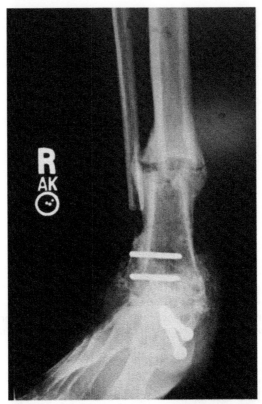

Fig. 10. Radiograph showing consolidation of the tibial regenerate and fusion of the ankle.

(**Table 1**). In all of these cases, it is important to optimize the patients by controlling their comorbidities and assessing their serum albumin for optimal healing. Discussion of the importance of smoking cessation and the effect of nicotine on bone healing is paramount. Obtaining a metabolic bone profile also is critical and this should include a comprehensive metabolic panel, vitamin D, thyroid-stimulating hormone, parathyroid hormone, calcium, and if necessary a bone density scan.

Table 1
Procedure and fixation options for different clinical scenarios

	Bone Loss <2 cm	Bone Loss >2 cm	Periprosthetic Infection	Minimal Ambulator
Indicated procedures	Bone grafting (femoral head, iliac crest)	Primary TC fusion with tibial lengthening Custom trabecular cage	Tissue samples, laboratory tests (C-reactive protein and interleukin-6), sonicate components, antibiotic spacer Primary septic fusion	Permanent antibiotic spacer
Fixation options	IM nail, plates, external fixation	External fixation, IM nail, plates	External fixation	Plate, IM nail

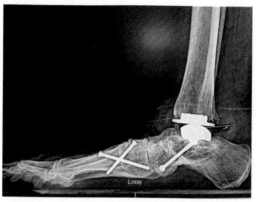

Fig. 11. Preoperative lateral radiograph of failed TAR with posterior extrusion of the polyethylene insert.

CASE PRESENTATIONS

The following case presentations illustrate some of the important aspects in procedural selection for these types of cases.

The first case is a 63-year-old woman who had stage IV posterior tibial tendon dysfunction. This initially was managed with a triple arthrodesis followed by placement of a total ankle implant and deltoid reconstruction when she was 57 years of age. The TAR surgery went well and she had no postoperative complications. She began to

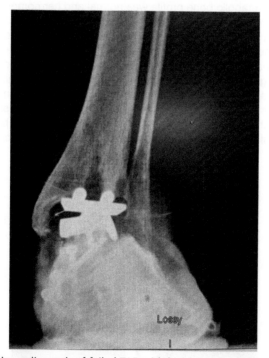

Fig. 12. Preoperative radiograph of failed TAR with lucency surrounding the tibial component and valgus angulation of the ankle.

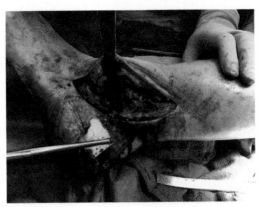

Fig. 13. Intraoperative photograph showing a segmental bone defect and broken polyethylene insert.

have pain and instability in her ankle approximately 4 years later. Her initial radiographs showed loosening of the implant with posterior extrusion of the polyethylene insert and valgus adaptation of her foot (**Figs. 11** and **12**). A computed tomography (CT) scan showed considerable osteolysis in the tibia. Due to the chamfer cuts necessary for this particular implant, it was difficult to determine the status of the talus (see **Fig. 11**). Conservative care failed and she did not want TAR revision, so the decision was made to perform an explant procedure. Based on the amount of bone loss and periprosthetic loosening, the decision was made to consider a TC fusion with distal lengthening. Her metabolic bone profile was normal and her comorbidities were well controlled. Her intraoperative bone and soft tissue cultures and bone biopsy specimens were negative for osteomyelitis. Intraoperatively, there was lucency around the tibial component, and the polypropylene was in 3 pieces. The segmental bone defect measured approximately 3.5 cm after the components and nonviable bone were removed (**Figs. 13** and **14**). The tibial cavity seen on CT was packed with cancellous chips and the ankle was temporarily reduced with a Steinmann pin. This placed the foot in a varus position because of the previous triple arthrodesis so a Gigli saw was utilized to osteotomize the midfoot and reduce it to a rectus position (**Figs. 15** and **16**). The incisions were closed and the circular fixator was applied. The midfoot

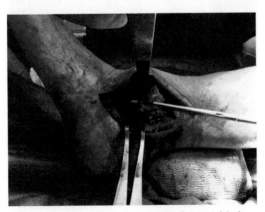

Fig. 14. Intraoperative photograph showing removal of nonviable bone.

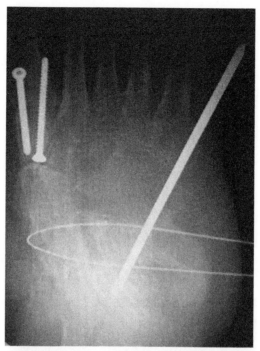

Fig. 15. Intraoperative anteroposterior foot radiograph of Gigli saw placement for a midfoot osteotomy.

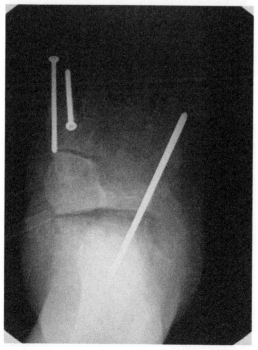

Fig. 16. Intraoperative anteroposterior foot radiograph after midfoot osteotomy.

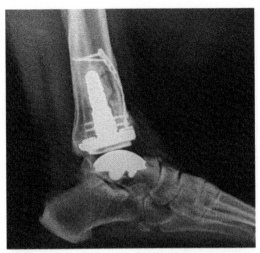

Fig. 17. Lateral radiograph with lucency at the anterior aspect of the tibial component and subsidence of the talus.

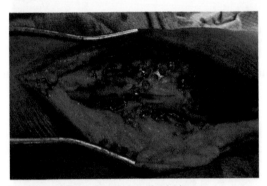

Fig. 18. Intraoperative photograph of anterior tibial plate.

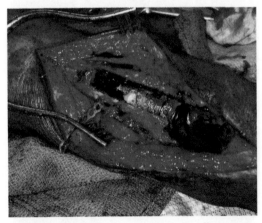

Fig. 19. Intraoperative photograph of the osteotomy to allow removal of the stemmed tibial component.

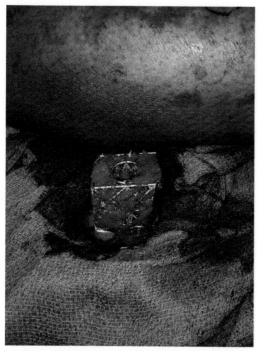

Fig. 20. Intraoperative photograph of the custom trabecular cage packed with autograft.

was fixated with a bent wire technique and the foot plate was compressed to the distal tibial ring to accomplish compression of the tibiocalcaneal fusion. The distal tibial corticotomy then was performed for eventual lengthening of the tibia. The latency period was 14 days and distraction began at 0.5 mm per day rather than 1 mm per day due to concerns with previous surgery of her ankle. Distraction continued until appropriate length was achieved, and the external fixator was not removed until consolidation of the regenerate was visualized on radiographs.

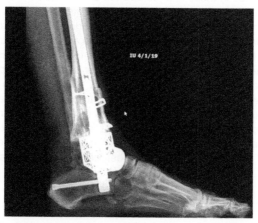

Fig. 21. Lateral radiograph of TAR explant with trabecular metal cage and IM nail 8 months postoperatively.

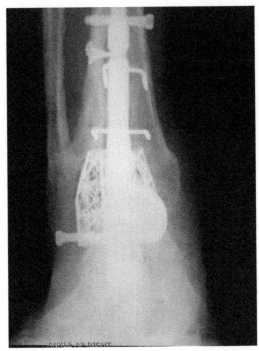

Fig. 22. Radiograph at 8 months postoperatively of total ankle explant with custom trabecular cage and IM nail.

The second case involves a 56-year-old woman who had a previous ankle fracture with eventual posttraumatic arthritis. She had a TAR when she was 51 years old. She began to have pain in the ankle approximately 3 years later that did not respond to conservative treatments. Her lateral radiograph showed radiolucency around the tibial component anteriorly and failure of the polyethylene insert. There also was subsidence of the talus (**Fig.17**). A CT was obtained to better assess the amount of bone loss. Based on the changes in these images and the significant bone loss in the tibia, the decision was made to consider a custom trabecular metal cage with and IM nail. Initial laboratory tests, including CBC with differential, sedimentation rate, and C-reactive protein, were within normal limits and her soft tissue and bone cultures were negative for infection. Her bone biopsy also was negative for osteomyelitis. This case was complicated by the inability to remove the modular stem of the implant without windowing the stem out from the anterior tibia (**Figs. 18** and **19**). The preexisting plate had a screw that was stripped and the plate had to be cut to gain access to remove the modular stem (see **Fig. 19**). Additional soft tissue and bone cultures were obtained along with bone biopsies. The custom cage was filled with autogenous bone graft from her proximal tibia as well as bone marrow aspirate and inset into the segmental bone defect with an IM nail (**Figs. 20–22**). Her postoperative course was uneventful and intraoperative cultures and biopsies were negative.

SUMMARY

Utilization of total joint replacement for end-stage ankle arthritis has gained popularity in recent years and has demonstrated excellent short-term and midterm outcomes in many patients. Revision components have been developed to handle those implants that have failed as a result of loosening of the components of the implant. Total ankle explant techniques also have been developed for those circumstances where conversion to a fusion or a permanent spacer is necessary. In the presence of infection and bone loss, there are techniques and fixation options available to improve outcomes in these difficult and complex cases.

REFERENCES

1. Vakhshori V, Sabour AF, Alluri RK, et al. Patient and practice trends in total ankle replacement and tibiotalar arthrodesis in the United States from 2007-2013. J Am Acad Orthop Surg 2019;27(2):e77–84.
2. Labek G, Thaler M, Janada W, et al. Revision rates after total joint replacement: cumulative results from worldwide register dataset. J Bone Joint Surg Br 2011; 93(3):293–7.
3. Labek G, Klaus H, Schlichtherle R, et al. Revision rates after total ankle arthroplasty in sample-based clinical studies and national registries. Foot Ankle Int 2011;32:7540–5.
4. Spirt A, Assal M, Hansen ST. Complicaitons and failure after total ankle arthroplasty. J Bone Joint Surg Am 2004;86-A:1172–8.
5. Gurney B. Leg length discrepancy. Gait Posture 2002;15(2):195–206.
6. Pyevich MT, Saltzman CL, Callaghan JJ, et al. Total ankle arthroplasty: a unique design. Two to twelve year follow-up. J Bone Joint Surg Am 1998;80(10):1410–20.
7. Knecht SI, Estin M, Callaghan JJ, et al. The Agility total ankle arthroplasty. Seven to sixteen -year follow-up. J Bone Joint Surg Am 2004;86-A(6):1161–71.
8. Unger AS, Clugis AE, Mow CS, et al. Total ankle arthroplasty in rheumatoid arthritis: a long tern follow-up study. Foot Ankle Int 1998;8:173.
9. Su EP, Kahn B, Flggle MP. Total ankle replacement in patients with rheumatoid arthritis. Clin Orthop Relat Res 2004;424:32–8.
10. Pilliar RM, Lee JM, Maniatopoulos C. Observations on the effect of movement on bone ingrowth into porous-surfaced implants. Clin Orthop Relat Res 1986;208: 108–13.
11. Jasty M, Bragdon C, Burke D, et al. In vivo skeletal responses to porous surfaced implants subjected to small induced motions. J Bone Joint Surg Am 1997;79(5): 707–14.
12. Kitaoka HB. Fusion techniques for failed total ankle arthroplasty. Semin Arthroplasty 1992;3:51–7.
13. Masquelet AC, Fitoussi F, Beque T, et al. Reconstruction of the long bones by the induced membrane and spongy autograft. Ann Chir Plast Esthet 2000;45(3): 346–53.
14. Carlsson AS, Montgomery F, Besjakov J. Arthrodesis of the ankle secondary to replacement. Foot Ankle Int 1998;19:240–5.
15. Doets HC, Zurcher AW. Salvage arthrodesis for failed total ankle arthroplasty. Clinical outcome and influence of method of fixation on union rate in 18 ankles followed for 3-12 years. Acta Orthop 2010;81(1):142–7.
16. Jeng CL, Campbell JT, Tang EY, et al. Tibiocalcaneal arthrodesis with bulk femoral head allograft for salvage of large defects in the ankle. Foot Ankle Int 2013;34(9):1256–66.
17. Bussewitz B, DeVries JG, Dujela M, et al. Retrograde intramedullary nail with femoral head allograft for large deficit tibiocalcaneal arthrodesis. Foot Ankle Int 2014;7:706–11.

18. Clements JR, Carpenter BB, Pourciau JK. Treating segmental bone defects: a new technique. J Foot Ankle Surg 2008;47(4):350–6.

19. Henricson A, Rydholm U. Use of trabecular metal implant in ankle arthrodesis after failed total ankle replacement: a short-term follow up of 13 patients. Acta Orthop 2010;81(6):745–7.

20. Mulhem JL, Protzman NM, White AM, et al. Salvage of failed total ankle replacement using a custom titanium truss. J Foot Ankle Surg 2016;55(4):868–73.

21. Ostermann P, Haase N, Rubberdt A, et al. Management of a long segmental defect at the proximal metaphyseal junction of the tibia using a cylindrical titanium mesh cage. J Orthop Trauma 2002;16:597–601.

22. Attias NA, Lindsey RW. Management of large segmental tibial defects using a cylindrical mesh cage. Clin Orthop Relat Res 2006;450:259–66.

23. Carlsson AS. Unsuccessful use of a titanium mesh cage in ankle arthrodesis: a report on three cases operated on due to a failed ankle replacement. J Foot Ankle Surg 2008;47:337–42.

24. Bullens P, de Waal Malefit M, Louwerens JW. Conversion of failed ankle arthroplasty to an arthrodesis. Technique using an arthrodesis nail and a cage filled with morsellized bone graft. Foot Ankle Surg 2010;16(2):101–4.

25. Chappell TM, Ebert CC, McCann KM, et al. Distal tibial distraction osteogenisis-an alternative approach to addressing limb length discrepancy with concurrent hindfoot and ankle reconstruction. J Orthop Surg Res 2019;14:244.

26. Rochman R, Jackson H, Aldae O. Tibiocalcaneal arthrodesis using the Ilizarov technique in the presence of bone loss and infection of the talus. Foot Ankle Int 2008;29(10):1001–8.

27. Sakurakichi K, Tsuchiya H, Uehara K, et al. Ankle arthrodesis combined with tibial lengthening using the Ilizarov apparatus. J Orthop Sci 2003;8(1):20–5.

28. McCoy TH, Goldman V, Fragomen AT, et al. Circular external fixator-assisted ankle arthrodesis following failed total ankle arthoplasty. Foot Ankle Int 2012;33(11):947–55.

29. Rabinovich RV, Haleem AM, Rozbruch SR. Complex ankle arthrodesis: review of the literature. World J Orthop 2015;6(8):602–13.

30. Lenarz C, Bledsoe G, Watson JT. Circular external fixation frames with divergent half pins: a pilot biomechanical study. Clin Orthop Relat Res 2008;466:2933–9.

31. Bronson DG, Samchukov ML, Birch JG, et al. Stability of external circular fixation. A multi-variable biomechnical analysis. Clin Biomech 1998;13:441–8.

32. Cierny G, Mader JT, Penninck JJ. A clinical staging system for adult osteomyelitis. Clin Orthop Relat Res 2003;414:7–24.

33. Ferrao P, Myerson MS, Schuberth JM, et al. Cement spacer as definitive management for post-operative ankle infection. Foot Ankle Int 2012;33(3):173–8.

34. Elmarsafi T, Oliver NG, Steinberg JS, et al. Long-term outcomes of permanent spacers in the infected foot. J Foot Ankle Surg 2017;56(2):287–90.

Revision of Malaligned Lapidus and Nonunited Lapidus

Donald E. Buddecke Jr, DPM[a],*, Eric R. Reese, DPM[b],
Ryan D. Prusa, DPM, PGY1[b]

KEYWORDS

• Lapidus • Bunionectomy • Arthrodesis

KEY POINTS

• Lapidus arthrodesis.
• Lapidus complications.
• Nonunion after Lapidus.
• Malunion after Lapidus.

INTRODUCTION

Correction of hallux valgus deformities has been evolving for decades. This stems from advancing knowledge of the entire triplane deformity and with development of superior fixation constructs. Correction of this deformity has typically been done by addressing the transverse plane. Various osteotomies have been devised for this purpose. This is logical, as this is the most severe abnormality visualized in this triplane problem. Attention to the sagittal plane component is not new. This is typically discussed as hypermobility of the first ray and subsequent dorsal and plantar motion in the sagittal plane. Progression of treatment started to migrate proximally to address this instability and also address the transverse plane. More recently, attention to the frontal plane deformity has gained popularity. The procedure that allows triplane correction is arthrodesis of the first tarsometatarsal (TMT) joint. Arthrodesis of the first TMT joint was first described in 1911[1] but was really popularized in 1934 by Paul Lapidus.[2] Now commonly bearing his name, this procedure continues to gain popularity. Understanding the mechanics of the first ray and entire medial column certainly drives this transition. Also, the better options for stable fixation make this a viable alternative for various hallux valgus deformities.

[a] Private Practice, PC, 18010 R Plaza, Omaha, NE 68135, USA; [b] Unitypoint Health - Iowa Methodist Medical Center, 1200 Pleasant Street, Des Moines, IA 50309, USA
* Corresponding author.
E-mail address: debuddecke@yahoo.com

Clin Podiatr Med Surg 37 (2020) 505–520
https://doi.org/10.1016/j.cpm.2020.03.010
0891-8422/20/© 2020 Elsevier Inc. All rights reserved.

Typically indicated for more severe deformities with associated instability, the Lapidus procedure is now being done on less pronounced deformities. The rationale is that the deformity can be corrected at its apex with more definitive correction. Additionally, this procedure can address all components of the deformity. The downside is generally a longer recovery time and possibly more complications. The most problematic complication after any hallux valgus surgery is recurrence. This remains a big concern with the Lapidus bunionectomy procedure. Additionally, one must worry about nonunion and malunion at the fusion site. These can be equally frustrating.

MALUNION

Malunion of a Lapidus procedure can present in a variety of ways. Some of these malunions are a result of placement in the less than ideal position, as this a relatively difficult procedure. In fact, Sangeorzan and Hansen stated "the relatively high incidence of failures can be attributed both to the technical complexity of the procedure and to the learning curve involved."[3] Trying to dial in the exact anatomic position is difficult in a patient who is a lying on the operating table. Later weight bearing of the patient can expose these less than ideal positions. At times, this is only 1° or 2° shy of perfection, and this lack of perfection is only exacerbated as the patient returns to his or her everyday activities. These patients had developed a triplane deformity prior to any surgical procedure. Consequently, it is not uncommon for some aspect of the deformity to return. The goal is to alter what the patient was born with and what has adapted over time and provide a stable construct that will last a lifetime. Continued research has helped guide these surgical techniques, but the procedure still requires the art (which is less than perfect) to finish the task on the operating table. Consequently, malunion can present as recurrence or undercorrection, elevation of the first metatarsal, excessive shortening, overcorrection, excessive plantarflexion of the first metatarsal, and lack of correction in the frontal plane.

UNDERCORRECTION/RECURRENCE

The most common malunion that occurs is actually recurrence of the deformity. Recurrence will vary with technique but has been reported to range from 3.2% to 60%[4,5] This can be a consequence of several factors. However, not gaining complete correction and fusion of the first TMT with widened intermetatarsal (IM) angle can present as a true malunion (**Fig. 1**). Different joint preparation techniques are available, including curettage and wedge resection. With either technique, the goal is to restore the first ray back to a normal position in all planes. If the IM angle is not completely corrected, the resulting fusion can be problematic. This can lead to difficulty in hallux valgus angle (HVA) reduction, and recurrence can develop. Another possibility is malunion in the frontal plane. If protonation of the first ray is present and correction is not performed, residual deformity can lead to recurrence. Much has been studied about the appearance of the tibial sesamoid position (TSP) and persistence of a round lateral first metatarsal head on AP radiographs when frontal plane deformity is not addressed.[4,6,7] The issue when not addressing the frontal plane is the lack of proper reduction of the sesamoids. Often, the sesamoids are not translated in relation to the first metatarsal, but the valgus position of the first metatarsal gives the appearance of a lateral deviation of the sesamoids. So, lack of frontal plane correction can lead to the sesamoids exerting a valgus pull on the hallux, leading to recurrence. However, in more severe deformities, the sesamoid can be translated in relation to the first metatarsal. A sesamoid axial view can demonstrate the tibial sesamoid sitting under or lateral to the median cristae (**Figs. 2 and 3**). As a result, many have stressed the

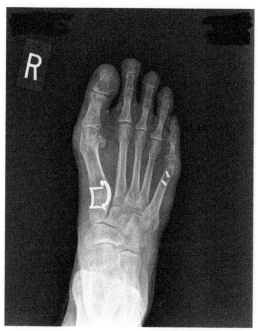

Fig. 1. Radiograph demonstrating malunited first ray after incomplete reduction of inter-metatarsal angle.

importance of complete triplane correction to prevent recurrence and demonstrated a recurrence rate of only 3.2% when this is accomplished.[4] Shibuya and colleagues[5] noted that the tibial sesamoid position was the only factor associated with recurrence. When the postoperative TSP was greater than 4, recurrence rate was about 50%. When postoperative TSP was greater than 5, the recurrence rate was about 60%. IM angle and HVA were not factors that led to recurrence in their study. Others have also attributed the lack of normalized TSP as a major factor with recurrence[8–10]

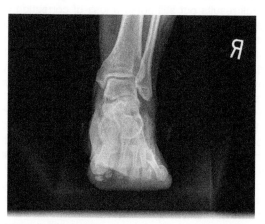

Fig. 2. Sesamoid axial view with frontal plane rotation and sesamoids remaining in normal position with regards to median cristae.

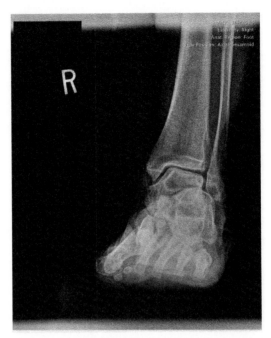

Fig. 3. Sesamoid axial view with lateral translation of sesamoids past median cristae.

Other overall foot structure issues can impact recurrence. The presence of metatarsus adductus has been shown to have higher recurrence rates.[11] Aiyer and colleagues[11] demonstrated a recurrence rate of 28.9% in the presence of metatarsus adductus and only 15.2% in those without metatarsus adductus (**Fig. 4**).

Despite successful fusion of the first TMT, there can be additional instability at the intercuneiform joint. This can lead to excessive force at this area, and an increase in the intermetatarsal angle can occur. Galli and colleagues[12] describe a technique using an additional screw from the first metatarsal base into the middle cuneiform to provide additional fixation and reduce hypermobility in the sagittal plane.[12] Another study revealed good overall results but still noted a loss of correction of the IM angle of 1.5°, HVA of 2.9°, and tibial sesamoid position of 0.8 positions with the use of a screw from the first metatarsal into middle cuneiform. These authors also compared results with the addition of 1 to 2 intermetatarsal screws and noticed slightly less recurrence with this construct.[13] This intercuneiform instability is not necessarily the cause of the recurrence but allows a slightly widened IM angle to occur. The recurrence is secondary to those factors previously discussed.

Revision bunion surgery is not a new concept. In the case of undercorrection or recurrence, multiple options are available. If the fusion has healed, any osteotomy with realignment to reduce the IM angle can be performed. The location of this osteotomy depends on the amount of correction that is needed. Distal osteotomies will lead to some additional shortening, as will any closing wedge osteotomy done more proximally. Opening wedge osteotomies are an option if maintaining length is a necessity. This can include various bone grafting, especially if multiple planes of correction are needed. It is imperative to assess the reason for the recurrence. If one does not address these reasons, such as persistent frontal plane problems, additional recurrence is all but guaranteed (**Fig. 5**).

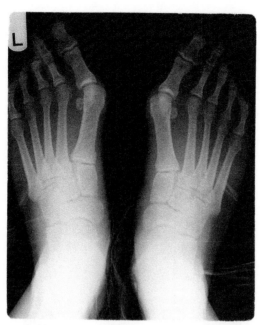

Fig. 4. Hallux valgus deformity with associated metatarsus adductus deformity. Notice the significant hallux valgus deformity but minimal increase in intermetatarsal angle. This limits the amount of correction that is available.

ELEVATION OF THE FIRST METATARSAL

Elevation of the first metatarsal is usually a result of poor positioning at the time of the procedure. However, weight bearing too early or with inadequate fixation can lead to adaptive elevation while the fusion construct is malleable. Attention to detail at the time of fusion can help mitigate this problem. When wedge resection is performed, the bone at the plantar portion of the joint is often difficult to remove. If left in place, the first metatarsal will be dorsally angulated. Additionally, care must be taken while making the wedge resection. There is a tendency to take less bone plantarly as one advanced the saw distally. The wedge should be assessed once it is removed. Similar problems can occur with curettage. If all cartilage is not removed from the plantar portion of the joint, abnormal dorsiflexion can occur in the final fusion construct. The first TMT joint has about twice the depth as width, making the deeper portion of the joint harder to assess. Malunion of the first metatarsal in an elevated position is not generally studied. However, Myerson[14] did report a rate of 9% elevated first ray after Lapidus arthrodesis (**Figs. 6 and 7**).

Dorsiflexion of the hallux at the first MTPJ at the time of provisional fixation can help position the first metatarsal adequately in the sagittal plane. Assessing this position with a true lateral view intraoperatively is vital. It is easy to angle the forefoot just a few degrees, which can give a false sagittal plane appearance. Simulating weight bearing with an even pressure to the forefoot while taking a true lateral radiograph is important for proper sagittal plane positioning.

A solid fixation construct can be advantageous at preventing first metatarsal elevation as the fusion site is healing. There is a trend for early weight bearing after these Lapidus procedures. If solid fixation is not present, elevation can develop prior to

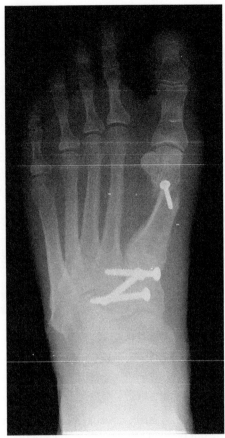

Fig. 5. A distal osteotomy was performed after recurrence of hallux valgus deformity from previous Lapidus arthrodesis. This patient also had additional stabilization of the intercuneiform joint.

this fusion becoming stiff. Dorsal, dorsomedial, and even medial plating is more common. Specific anatomic plates are readily available, including plantar positioned plates, providing an option of fixation on the tension side of the fusion site.

Additional fixation alterations have been adapted to help prevent dorsal elevation of the first metatarsal. Interfragmentary compression screws from the first metatarsal into the medial cuneiform is common. However, additional interfragmentary compression can be gained by placing a screw from the first metatarsal base into the middle cuneiform or into the second metatarsal base. This can give the advantage of additional stabilization in the transverse plane but also more stability in the sagittal plane. The sagittal plane position between the first and second rays is maintained with this construct until the fusion is solid. If complaints of excessive stiffness are noted after fusion is complete, the screw can be removed (**Figs. 8 and 9**).

Symptoms that are noted with an elevated first metatarsal can include lesser metatarsalgia or even hallux rigidus with jamming and the first MTPJ. If lesser metatarsalgia is noted, make sure this is related to first ray elevation and not excessive first metatarsal shortening. Attention to detail on the lateral radiograph is vital. Often, patients

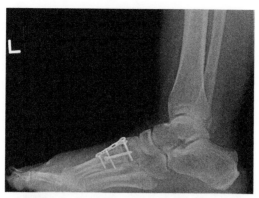

Fig. 6. Lapidus arthrodesis performed with interfragmentary screw and dorsal locking plate fixation. Notice the good anatomic alignment in the sagittal plane with the first metatarsal declination being parallel to the second metatarsal declination.

can stand in a slightly corrected position, giving a false appearance to the sagittal plane alignment of the first metatarsal.

Correction of an elevated first metatarsal can be relatively simple. An osteotomy made in the proximal portion of the bone with dorsally based wedge is common. Leaving the plantar cortex intact and using dorsal plate fixation lead to a stable osteotomy. The amount of correction can be dialed in, and revision of the fusion can be avoided.

Excessive Shortening

Another form of malunion is excessive shortening. Unless bone grafting is performed, some aspect of shortening will occur with any fusion procedure. Often curettage of the cartilage surfaces is done to minimize the shortening. When wedge resection is performed, it is usually done with as minimal of bone resection as possible. Several complications can present from excessive shortening, including lesser metatarsalgia, hallux interphalangeus, or lesser digital deformities. Sangeorzan and Hansen[3] reported an average shortening of 5.0 mm with the Lapidus procedure. Catanzariti and colleagues[15] reported an average shortening of 4.7 mm, while McInnes and

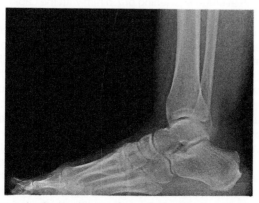

Fig. 7. Lateral radiograph after hardware removal secondary to infection. Notice the dorsal elevation of the first ray that occurred compared with **Fig. 6.**

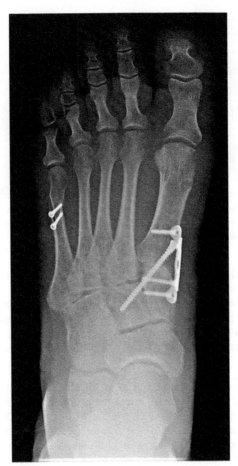

Fig. 8. Lapidus arthrodesis performed with interfragmentary screw from first metatarsal to the middle cuneiform and associated medial locking plate.

Bouché[16] reported an average shortening of 7.5 mm with the Lapidus procedure. One can see from this variation of shortening that surgical technique plays a significant role. If preoperative radiographs demonstrate an already shortened first ray or elongated second metatarsal, this will exaggerate the imbalance of the metatarsal parabola. Modifications can be implemented to maintain purchase if a shortened first ray is present prior to the Lapidus procedure. Slightly plantarflexing the first metatarsal on the cuneiform or inferiorly translating the first metatarsal on the cuneiform can help in many cases. Bone grafting to maintain length is also an option. However, it remains ideal to maintain a normal metatarsal parabola in place of these alterations. Lesser metatarsal osteotomies can also be performed (**Fig. 10**).

Assessing the symptoms from an excessively shortened first metatarsal is important to help determine the best plan for correction. Bone grafting to gain length can be done. Again, this can be done at the fusion site or slightly distal on the first metatarsal if one does not want to take down the fusion site. It is preferable to perform the osteotomy in metaphyseal bone. Alternatively, or in addition to bone grafting (in cases of excessive length discrepancy), shortening osteotomy of the second metatarsal or

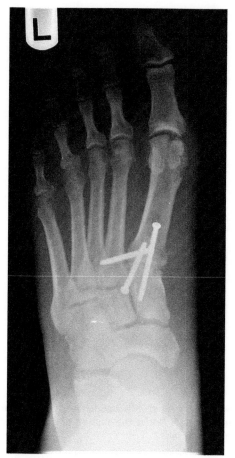

Fig. 9. Lapidus arthrodesis performed with standard cross-screws and associated screw from first metatarsal to the second metatarsal.

second and third metatarsals can be performed. Sangeorzan and Hansen demonstrated that 4 mm of lengthening can be gained with grafting.[3]

Plantarflexed First Ray

In an attempt to prevent dorsiflexion malunion, overplantarflexing the first metatarsal can overload the first MPJ, resulting in sesamoid pain. Excessive plantar wedge resection or excessive plantar translation can lead to first ray overload. The mobility between first and second metatarsals and the medial and middle cuneiforms can partially accommodate for this mishap. However, if one's Lapidus technique includes variations of stabilization between first and second metatarsal bases and/or stabilization at the intercuneiform area, less accommodative mobility is available. This can result in more sesamoid type pain.

Similar to the correction of an elevated first metatarsal, correction of a plantarflexed metatarsal is relatively simple. A dorsal closing wedge osteotomy can be made at a desired location on the metatarsal. Preferably, this is more proximal in metaphyseal bone, and the plantar cortex is left intact. The metatarsal is dorsiflexed, closing the

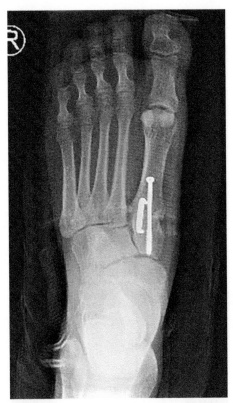

Fig. 10. Lapidus arthrodesis performed with wedge resection and stabilized with interfragmentary screw and staple fixation. Notice the amount of shortening of the first metatarsal in relation to the lesser metatarsals.

osteotomy site, and fixation is performed. This can be done with a dorsal plate or staple fixation.

OVERCORRECTION/NEGATIVE INTERMETATARSAL

Excessive closure of the IM angle can lead to a difficult malunion. This is not typical of curettage type techniques. Overzealous wedge resection can lead to a negative IM angle. Combining this overcorrection with additional soft tissue work at the MTPJ places the patient at a higher risk of hallux varus. Reported rates of hallux varus after Lapidus procedures is not abundant. However, there are reports of 10% to 16% rate of hallux varus after Lapidus arthrodesis.[17,18]

Addressing this complication may only require soft tissue work at the MTPJ. However, this can also be addressed with osteotomies of the proximal phalanx of the great toe. If the deformity is more severe, a metatarsal osteotomy can be performed to normalize the IM angle. Distal or proximal osteotomies are available depending on the amount of correction needed (**Fig. 11**).

NONUNION

Nonunion after any arthrodesis procedure is always a leading risk. This remains true for Lapidus arthrodesis. Rates of nonunion range from 0% to 12%[16,19–22] The specific

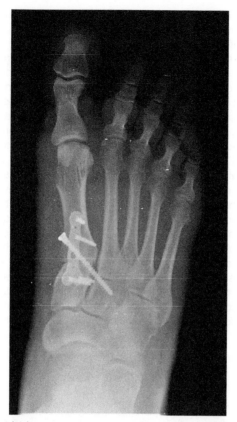

Fig. 11. Radiograph with almost negative IM angle and early start of hallux varus deformity.

joint mechanics, the lever arm that is present, and the push to bear weight early after these procedures all play a role. Three main factors that continue to be described as a concern include joint preparation techniques, the fixation construct used, and early weight bearing. These are the surgeon factors. There are patient factors as well. Overall health status including diabetes, smoking, and vitamin D and calcium levels will play a role. Patient compliance will always be a concern.

Joint preparation involves either planal resection of the joint surfaces or curettage. Obvious planal resection provides great bleeding bone for healing purposes, but it can be difficult getting perfect positioning and can lead to excessive shortening. Curettage was adopted to help minimize some of these issues. However, the concerns with curettage include the potential for higher nonunion as one attempts to leave the subchondral plate in place. Prissel and colleagues[22] did reveal a better union rate with planal resection (97.8%) when compared with curettage (91.5%). However, the curettage technique has been shown to have low nonunion rates.[23] Patel and colleagues [23] reported a nonunion rate of 5.3% in 227 patients while using curettage for joint preparation. A similar report showed 5% nonunion rate with curettage.[20] This was a much larger study with 599 patients. Conversely, utilizing planal resection does not guarantee successful union. A rate of nonunion of 8.3% has been reported in the recent literature after planal resection.[24] The amount of shortening after planal resection versus curettage was evaluated.[25] Planal resection resulted in 3.14 mm of shortening compared to just 0.86 mm with curettage. IM correction was statistically similar, and nonunions were reported. Understanding the potential risks with each technique can help mitigate some of the complications.

The hardware utilized for Lapidus arthrodesis continues to evolve in an attempt to prevent nonunion complications. The modern era started with cross-screw fixation. The first screw is placed from the dorsal first metatarsal and driven into the plantar medial cuneiform in a lag screw fashion. A second screw is placed from dorsal aspect of medial cuneiform and driven into the plantar first metatarsal base to act as an anti-rotational screw (**Fig. 12**). Donnenwerth and colleagues[20] performed a systemic review of curettage technique with cross-screw fixation. They found 5% nonunion rate. A trend toward a more stable construct has evolved to allow earlier weight bearing. Interfragmentary screw with locking plate construct was shown to be superior when compared to cross-screws and an interfragmentary screw with a nonlocking plate.[22] Fixation on the tension side of the fusion construct has been evaluated.[26–28] A plantar interfragmentary screw with medial locking plate revealed a union in 86 of 88 feet.[26] Cadaveric studies have also been performed showing superiority of plantar plating.[27,28] Additional research has included stabilization from the first metatarsal to the middle cuneiform and first metatarsal to second metatarsal.[13] The goal was to provide a more rigid construct to reduce nonunion but also reduce recurrence. A cadaver study demonstrated that standard 2-point fixation of the first tarsometatarsal joint reduced first ray motion by 40.8%. Adding additional fixation from the first metatarsal into the middle cuneiform reduced the motion by 58.1%. The authors noted that there

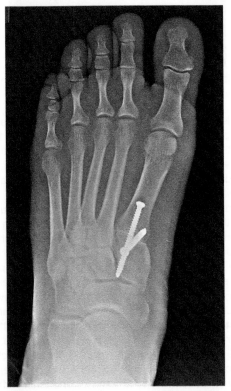

Fig. 12. Lapidus arthrodesis performed with curettage and standard 2 screw fixation.

was still 3.1 mm of motion available to allow midfoot compensation..[12] A study by Barp and colleagues[29] compared nonunion rates of fixation techniques. These authors found nonunion rates of 9% for crossing screw fixation, 5% for interfragmentary screw with locking plate, and 2% for locking plate fixation with integrated compression screw within the plate. Mallet and colleagues[24] investigated the rate of nonunion when using staple fixation. They noted an 8.3% (3 of 36) nonunion rate.

Early weightbearing has been a trend in the post-operative course after Lapidus bunionectomy. More stable constructs at the fusion site allow patients to be bearing weight as soon as immediately after surgery. In a systematic review by Crowell and colleagues,[30] 443 arthrodesis cases were analyzed. Early weight bearing was defined as less than 2 weeks postoperatively. They found a total nonunion rate of 3.61%. In a multicenter study by Ray and colleagues,[4] most patients were allowed to be fully weight bearing as tolerated in a boot walker the day of surgery. A symptomatic nonunion rate of 1.6% was reported. In another multicenter study of 80 patients, a 100% union rate was noted, with a mean time to weight bearing of 14.8 days.[19]

Diagnosis of nonunion starts with plain radiographs. Lucency at the fusion site and hardware failure are often noted. Some cases are easily diagnosed (**Fig. 13**). Signs of lucency with or without hardware failure in addition to symptoms at the fusion site are concerns. At times, there are symptoms at the fusion site but no clear-cut sign of

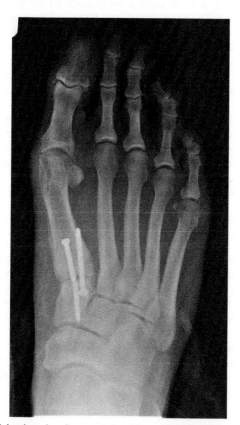

Fig. 13. Lucency and broken hardware at Lapidus arthrodesis site indicating nonunion. Notice the resultant increase in IM angle and recurrence of hallux valgus angle.

nonunion. It may be difficult to distinguish painful scar tissue or implant irritation from delayed union or nonunion. Computed tomography is vital is these cases.

In some cases of nonunion the patient will be asymptomatic. Surgery is not indicated in these patients. If a patient is symptomatic, then revision surgery should be considered. The revision needs to focus on the factors that lead to lack of healing. Poor fixation construct, poor patient biology (eg, diabetes, smoking, and vitamin D deficiency), and poor compliance need to be addressed. If a significant amount of shortening will occur after removal of the un-united portion of bone, bone grafting should be planned. Multiple options are available including precut tricortical bone blocks, autogenous bone grafts, or a combination. Augmenting options including bone marrow aspirate, platelet rich plasma, and amniotic cells can be valuable tools. Revision surgery always has increased risks, but success is possible.

The largest published case series by Hamilton and colleagues[31] evaluated rate of union after revision Lapidus arthrodesis. Seventeen cases of revisional bone block TMT arthrodesis were evaluated. Bone stimulators were used immediately postoperatively in 13 patients. Postoperative course included not bearing weight for 6 weeks in a short leg cast with progression to a walking boot for 4 weeks if radiographic consolidation was noted. Patients were transitioned to regular shoes at an average of 10 weeks. A total of 14 (82%) patients went on to union, and 3 (18%) had recurrent nonunion. In 2 of the 3 recurrent nonunions, the patient remained symptomatic at the time of the study. The other patient underwent an additional revision surgery, and union was achieved. The study also found that smoking was a statistically significant predictor of nonunion. In a study looking at the nonunion rate after modified Lapidus arthrodesis, Patel and colleagues[23] briefly described completing revisional surgery on 7 nonunions following Lapidus bunionectomy. Each case had autogenous bone graft from either the iliac crest, distal tibia, or calcaneus. Six of the 7 cases went on to union. The remaining patient was asymptomatic and did not undergo additional surgery.

Bone graft alternatives have been used for Lapidus nonunions. A case study was described where a custom 3-dimensionally printed titanium truss implant was used to fill a large osseous defect after a septic nonunion.[32] Because of the amount of bone that needed to be removed, a 3-dimensionally printed truss was manufactured to fill the void. The patient went on to heal uneventfully. Cases such as this are not typical, but they demonstrate various alternatives for those unique cases with extensive bone loss.

DISCUSSION

The understanding of hallux valgus deformities continues to evolve. Various surgical procedures have been described over the last several decades. Arthrodesis of the first TMT joint seems to be a procedure that is utilized more frequently. This procedure offers the ability to correct minor to severe deformities. It also has the ability to gain triplane correction at the apex of the deformity. This procedure has its challenges. The learning curve is somewhat steep, and this is not an easy procedure. Complications will happen and range from nonunion to various alignment issues of the first ray. It is imperative to understand the variations in the deformity and properly diagnose problems when they develop. If done properly, successful outcomes are obtainable.

DISCLOSURE

The authors have nothing to disclose.

REFERENCES

1. Albrecht GH. The pathology and treatment of hallux valgus. Russk Vrach 1911; 10:11–9.
2. Lapidus PW. Operative correction of metatarsus varus primus in hallux valgus. Surg Gynecol Obstet 1934;58:183–91.
3. Sangeorzan B, Hansen S. Modified Lapidus procedure for hallux valgus. Foot Ankle 1992;13:107–15.
4. Ray J, Koay J, Dayton P, et al. Multicenter early radiographic outcomes of triplanar tarsometatarsal arthrodesis with early weightbearing. Foot Ankle Int 2019;40: 955–60.
5. Shibuya N, Kyprios EM, Panchani PN, et al. Factors associated with early loss of hallux valgus correction. J Foot Ankle Surg 2018;57:236–40.
6. Dayton P, Kauwe M, DiDomenico L, et al. Quantitative analysis of the degree of frontal rotation required to anatomically align the first metatarsal phalangeal joint during modified tarsal-metatarsal arthrodesis without capsular balancing. J Foot Ankle Surg 2016;55:220–5.
7. Dayton P, Carvalho S, Dayton M. Comparison of radiographic measurements before and after triplane tarsometatarsal arthrodesis for hallux valgus. J Foot Ankle Surg 2020;59:291–7.
8. Sammarco GJ, Idusyi OB. Complications after surgery of the hallux. Clin Orthop Relat Res 2001;391:58–71.
9. Okuda R, Kinoshita M, Morikawa J, et al. Distal soft tissue procedure and proximal metatarsal osteotomy in hallux valgus. Clin Orthop Relat Res 2000;379: 209–17.
10. Okuda R, Kinoshita M, Yasuda T, et al. Postoperative incomplete reduction of the sesamoids as a risk factor for recurrence of hallux valgus. J Bone Joint Surg Am 2009;91:1637–45.
11. Aiyer A, Shub J, Shariff R, et al. Radiographic recurrence of deformity after hallux valgus surgery in patients with metatarsus adductus. Foot Ankle Int 2015;37: 165–71.
12. Galli MM, McAlister JE, Berlet GC, et al. Enhanced Lapidus arthrodesis: crossed screw technique with middle cuneiform fixation further reduces sagittal mobility. J Foot Ankle Surg 2015;54:437–40.
13. Langan TM, Greschner JM, Brandao RA, et al. Maintenance of correction of the modified lapidus procedure with a first metatarsal to intermediate cuneiform cross-screw technique. Foot Ankle Int 2019.
14. Myerson M. Metatarsocuneiform arthrodesis for treatment of hallux valgus and metatarsus primus varus. Orthopedics 1990;13:1025–31.
15. Catanziriti AR, Mendocino RW, Lee MS, et al. The modified Lapidus arthrodesis: a retrospective analysis. J Foot Ankle Surg 1999;38:322–32.
16. McInnes BD, Bouche RT. Critical evaluation of modified Lapidus procedure. J Foot Ankle Surg 2001;40:71–90.
17. Kopp FJ, Patel MM, Levine DS, et al. The modifed Lapidus procedure for hallus valgus: a clinical and radiographic analysis. Foot Ankle Int 2005;26:913–7.
18. Mauldin DM, Sanders M, Whitmer MW. Correction of hallux valgus with metatarsocuneiform stabilization. Foot Ankle 1990;11:59–66.
19. Blitz NM, Lee T, Williams SK, et al. Early weight bearing after modified lapidus arthrodesis: a multicenter review of 80 cases. J Foot Ankle Surg 2010;49:357–62.
20. Donnenwerth MP, Borkosky SL, Abicht BP, et al. Rate of nonunion after first metatarsal-cuneiform arthrodesis using joint curettage and two crossed

compression screw fixation: a systematic review. J Foot Ankle Surg 2011;50: 707–9.

21. Lagaay PM, Hamilton GA, Ford LA, et al. Rates of revision surgery using chevron-austin osteotomy, Lapidus arthrodesis, and closing base wedge osteotomy for correction of hallux valgus deformity. J Foot Ankle Surg 2008;47:267–72.

22. Prissel MA, Hyer CF, Grambart ST, et al. A multicenter, retrospective study of early weightbearing for modified Lapidus arthrodesis. J Foot Ankle Surg 2016;55: 226–9.

23. Patel S, Ford LA, Etcheverry J, et al. Modified Lapidus arthrodesis: rate of nonunion in 227 cases. J Foot Ankle Surg 2004;43:37–42.

24. Mallette JP, Glenn CL, Glod DJ. The incidence of nonunion after Lapidus arthrodesis using staple fixation. J Foot Ankle Surg 2014;53:303–6.

25. Boffeli TJ, Hyllengren SB. Can we abandon saw wedge resection in Lapidus fusion? A comparative study of joint preparation techniques regarding correction of deformity, union rate, and preservation of 1st ray length. J Foot Ankle Surg 2019;58:1118–24.

26. Cottom JM,, Vora AM. Fixation of Lapidus arthrodesis with a plantar interfragmentary screw and medial locking plate: a report of 88 cases. J Foot Ankle Surg 2013; 52:465–9.

27. Klos K, Simons P, Hajduk AS, et al. Plantar vs dorsomedial locked plating for Lapidus arthrodesis: a biomechanical comparison. Foot Ankle Int 2011;32:1081–5.

28. Roth KE, Peters J, Schmidtmann I, et al. Intraosseous fixation compared to plantar plate fixation for first metatarsocuneiform arthrodesis: a cadaveric biomechanical analysis. Foot Ankle Int 2014;35:1209–16.

29. Barp EA, Erickson JG, Smith HL, et al. Evaluation of fixation techniques for metatarsocuneiform arthrodesis. J Foot Ankle Surg 2017;56:468–73.

30. Crowell A, Van JC, Meyr AJ. Early weightbearing after arthrodesis of the first metatarsal-medial cuneiform joint: a systemic review of the incidence of nonunion. J Foot Ankle Surg 2018;57:1204–6.

31. Hamilton GA, Mullins S, Schuberth JM, et al. Revision Lapidus arthrodesis: rate of union in 17 cases. J Foot Ankle Surg 2007;46:447–50.

32. So E, Mandas VH, Hlad L. Large osseous defect reconstruction using a custom three-dimensional printed titanium truss implant. J Foot Ankle Surg 2018;57: 196–204.

Revision of Recurrent Neuromas

Katherine Frush, DPM*, Amanda Niester, BS, DPM

KEYWORDS

- Interdigital neuroma • Recurrent neuroma • Revision • Surgical treatment
- Neurectomy • Nerve transposition • Conduit

KEY POINTS

- Recurrence is related to the misunderstanding of cause, misdiagnosis, or improper primary treatment, either by treatment option or technique.
- Traditionally revision surgery is done by plantar excisional approach because of increased visualization.
- Newer techniques including use of conduits or nerve transposition may be used for primary neuromas or may be used for neuroma recurrence.

INTRODUCTION

A neuroma is an enlarged, irritated nerve found in the interspace of the toes, most commonly in the third followed by the second interspace,[1] which presents with immense pain in the forefoot. One of the first clinical representations of this syndrome dates back to 1876 when Morton[2] described a "peculiar and painful affection of the foot, localized in the fourth metatarsophalangeal articulation." Although this syndrome has been present for a long time, the pathology of its occurrence is still not definitive, which makes it challenging to treat. A few theorized causes include ischemia[3] and nerve entrapment.[4,5] Another challenge is that neuromas are one of the many diagnoses that are blanketed into metatarsalgia, so it is important to perform adequate tests to confirm a neuroma and rule out other possibilities. When a neuroma is diagnosed and treatment begins, it most often starts with conservative methods. However, roughly 80% of patients do not get sufficient relief with conservative treatment and proceed to surgical interventions.[6] Furthermore, after excision, pain persists 20% to 82% of the time.[7,8] This paper reviews the revisional surgeries for the recurrent neuroma; but more importantly, it discusses the opportunity to reduce recurrence through the understanding of neuroma biology, diagnosis, and treatment options.

Des Moines University, College of Podiatric Medicine and Surgery, 3200 Grand Avenue, Des Moines, IA 50312, USA
* Corresponding author.
E-mail address: katherine.frush@dmu.edu

Clin Podiatr Med Surg 37 (2020) 521–532
https://doi.org/10.1016/j.cpm.2020.03.007
0891-8422/20/© 2020 Elsevier Inc. All rights reserved.

BIOLOGY
Anatomy

The Morton neuroma is an enlarged common plantar digital nerve and is most commonly found in the third interspace, which is thought to be caused by the anatomic features. One factor is that in 66.2% of cases, there is a communicating branch between the third and fourth common plantar digital nerves that passes plantar to the fourth metatarsal. Another factor is the deep transverse metatarsal ligament. The nerve passes below the ligament, and because its anatomic position is just proximal to the metatarsal heads adjacent to the interspace, it has been suspected that the neuroma formation is caused by entrapment and/or mechanical forces in this area.[9] Nissen[3] recognizes other anatomic features that may play a role in the neuroma formation, including the third plantar digital artery, lumbrical to the fourth toe, transverse head of adductor hallucis, intermetatarsophalangeal bursa, and fat. Macroscopically, a neuroma appears thickened with amorphous material around it that adheres it to surrounding blood vessels and subcutaneous fat.[10]

Histology

Histologically, neuromas have been found to have abnormalities in the nerve, artery, and interstitium. Giannini and colleagues[10] find that nerves present with demyelination, edema, and fibrosis of the perineurium and epineurium. This study also shows that it is possible to find increased fibrotic and elastic fibers in the interstitium along with edema and degenerative changes. In vessels, proliferative changes are found in the muscular layer and adventitia. Other studies have found similar findings.[3,5,9,11] Nissen[3] believes that the vascular degeneration seen histologically, along with macroscopic findings, proves the theory that the painful neuroma forms secondary to this degeneration. Although the previously listed studies conclude that the histologic findings are unique to neuromas, a separate study compares the histologic findings of neuromas and intermetatarsal nerves from cadavers and finds degenerative nerve changes in both.[12] Note that there are histologic differences between primary and recurrent neuromas. Primary neuromas present with degenerative changes, whereas recurrent neuromas show proliferation.[13]

Repair After Excision

When a neuroma is excised, the proximal and distal ends react in unique ways to attempt to rejoin. This response is started by the nerve cell body in the dorsal root ganglion, which metabolizes rebuilding products that are sent to the site of excision through axoplasmic transport. Both ends continue with Wallerian degeneration, but the distal end degenerates further, leading to empty endoneurial tubes, whereas the proximal end develops budding axons with regenerating factors that seek the empty tubes of the distal nerve end to close the gap. If the proximal end fails to connect with the distal end, it can get stuck in the periphery. However, the need to repair the disrupted endoneurium drives the budding axons to continue searching for the distal end in a disorganized pattern, which leads to the formation of a stump neuroma.[14]

DIAGNOSIS

It is important to keep differentials in mind that may present similarly including neuropathic pain related to diabetes and hypothyroidism,[15] plantar plate tear, degenerative and inflammatory arthritis, stress fracture, Freiberg infarction, bursitis, fat pad atrophy, and transfer metatarsalgia.[6,16–18] The long list of differentials emphasizes the need for a thorough history, physical examination, and use of any necessary diagnostic tests.

Common subjective findings include discomfort when wearing shoes, especially high heels; a burning sensation and/or the feeling of a pebble in the affected interspace; and sudden pain when walking.[1,10,17,18] The pain is described as intermittently sharp or constantly aching.[19] Symptoms are usually relieved when the uncomfortable shoe is removed or walking is limited.

On physical examination, there should be limited dermatologic abnormalities, including no sign of infection.[2] Points of pain on palpation are found on the plantar aspect of the foot, just proximal to the metatarsal necks adjacent to the affected interspace along with distal radiation to the toes at times, suggesting a positive Tinel sign.[3,20] The Mulder test (**Fig. 1**) is performed by wrapping one hand around the foot so that your fingers squeeze the metatarsal heads together while the other hand squeezes the interspace from plantar to dorsal so that the mass is felt and at times a click is heard or felt.[21] The Gauthier test (**Fig. 2**), which is highly sensitive for nerve compression, is performed as well by squeezing the metatarsal heads together, similar to the Mulder method, and alternating active dorsiflexion and plantarflexion to assess pain symptoms. Pain should be present when toe is in dorsiflexed position and absent when plantarflexed.[4] It is always important to check the second and third interspaces for thorough evaluation. If suspicious of a plantar plate tear, it is also beneficial to assess for any malalignment of the symptomatic metatarsophalangeal joint and perform a drawer test to rule that out.[16]

Further tests are performed to aid in the diagnosis and localization of the neuroma. Lateral and anteroposterior radiographs do not diagnose a neuroma, but they rule out osseous or joint abnormalities that can cause metatarsalgia.[9,10,16,22] There has been debate on the usefulness of MRI and ultrasound. A study by Fazal and colleagues[23]

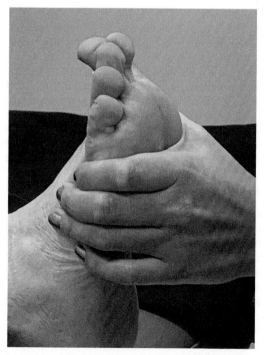

Fig. 1. Gauthier test.

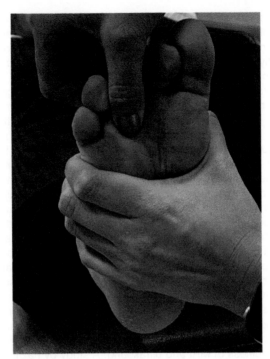

Fig. 2. Mulder compression test.

found MRI to present a neuroma as a bulbous, hypointense mass on T1 and T2 that is located plantarly in the intermetatarsal space. This study also found that MRI is a poor method of detecting neuromas smaller than 5 mm. The use of ultrasonography was also analyzed in this study and it was found that neuromas appear as ovoid, hypoechoic masses parallel to the long axis of the metatarsal. This method was found to have a 96% sensitivity of detecting neuromas, including those smaller than 5 mm.[23] Other studies also found ultrasound to be helpful because of the availability, higher sensitivity, and lower cost, and one even found it beneficial to detect the Mulder sign.[24,25] Steroid or nerve block injections have been found to be beneficial in diagnosing neuromas and plantar plate tears, a common differential.[16,20]

TREATMENT OPTIONS

It has been suggested that neuroma treatment should incorporate a treatment ladder. One study's ladder started with shoe modifications, then cortisone injection, and finally, excision. The authors allowed 3 months between each treatment to evaluate whether symptoms were satisfactorily relieved before moving up the ladder. With 85% of patients being satisfied with their overall treatment, only 21% went on to surgery.[1] This re-emphasizes that although neuromas are challenging to treat, conservative options do work at times, and this should be addressed with the patient. When deciding the appropriate treatment option, it is important to educate the patient on the possible procedures along with their success rates and risk of complications so that the option best suited for that individual is made. Along with shoe modifications and cortisone injections,[17,24,26] other conservative options include sclerosing injections[27–29] and physical therapy modalities.[30] When conservative options have failed, surgical options should be explored.

Surgical

The surgical options summarized next are used for primary and recurrent neuroma treatment. The technique used for initial may limit some of these options to primary surgery only.

- Endoscopic decompression[5]:
  - This addresses the entrapment of the nerve within the transverse intermetatarsal ligament.
  - Methods:
    - Make a dorsal incision and two plantar incisions, one being transverse at the web space, distal to the weightbearing surface, and the other more proximal to the weightbearing surface, at the level of the plantar arch.
    - Pass a cannula through the two plantar incisions, and use a 2.3-mm, 30° beveled scope for visualization.
    - Place the deep transverse metatarsal ligament into an optimum position using a metatarsal retractor in the dorsal portal.
    - Transect the ligament by inserting a curved blade into the cannula.
  - Results:
    - 86% of patients were found to have excellent or good results.
  - This is a good primary option to decompress the interspace but is not a great option if the neuroma was previously excised through a dorsal approach because the ligament will have already been transected.
- Neurectomy:
  - Dorsal approach:
    - The study by Gauthier[4] finds 83% of patients to have improvements after a longitudinal dorsal approach with plantar fascia release.
    - When combined, the two studies performed by Akermark and colleagues[22,31] find a significant increase in stump neuromas or missed neuromas in the dorsal group at 12%.
  - Plantar approach:
    - Nery and colleagues[32] perform a distal plantar transverse incision, which results in 89.4% of patients having good results all the way through the 7-year follow-up.
    - The combined studies by Akermark and colleagues[22,31] find 0% of the plantar group to have stump neuromas or missed nerve complications.
    - Faraj and Hosur[33] find complications including wound infection, hematoma, scar problems, and delayed return to weightbearing to be significantly higher in the plantar group. There is one patient that presents with recurrent pain in this group compared with none in the dorsal group.
  - It has been debated if one approach is more effective than the other, and although authors have their preferred methods, they have not been able to confirm a true superior treatment.
  - Neither the dorsal nor plantar approaches for excision have stood out as being the gold standard for neuroma treatment, so physicians have continued to seek ways to enhance the procedure.
- Nerve transposition:
  - Transposition into intermuscular septa[34]:
    - Methods:

- Using a dorsal approach, the deep transverse intermetatarsal ligament is transected to visualize the neuroma.
- The proper plantar digital nerves in that interspace are also transected, 5 mm distal to their bifurcation from the common digital nerve.
- Using suture material and a Keith needle, the proximal end of the excision is looped proximal and deep to be placed in the intermuscular space between the transverse head of the adductor hallucis and the interossei.
- The transposed nerve is then secured to the plantar skin.
  - Results:
    - At 1- and 6-month follow-ups: higher pain levels in the transposition group compared with the excision group.
    - At 36- to 48-month follow-up: the transposition group has a significantly lower pain level. The transposition group also reports better pain relief with 96% excellent and 4% good, whereas the excision group has 86% excellent and 14% fair.
  - Dorsal transposition[17,35]:
    - Methods:
      - Song and colleagues[35] perform neuroma resections through a dorsal approach along with transposition of the proximal end dorsally by securing it to the dorsal transverse ligament.
      - Vito and Talarico[17] perform a dorsal approach neuroma and dorsal transposition of the proximal end by securing it to the deep fascia of the adjacent metatarsal.
  - Vein transposition[36]:
    - The animal study shows that nerves transposed into a vein resist the abnormal patterns seen in stump neuromas, and instead they have a more organized endoneurial structure with minifascicles running in the same direction, along with a normal amount of myelinated axons and limited connective tissue formation.
    - None of the veins used in this study thrombosed.
    - Better fixation needs to be attained than what was done in the study, and the authors suggest epineural transmural stitches at the distal end of the nerve stump along with circular epineural stitches around the venotomy.
- Decompression and distal metatarsal osteotomy of second, third, and fourth metatarsals[18]:
  - Methods:
    - Create a dorsal portal at the level of the associated metatarsal heads using a beaver blade.
    - Enter the blade into the web space at a 45-degree angle to the metatarsal shaft, pointing distal and plantar toward the metatarsal neck.
    - Push the blade further distal, running parallel to the metatarsal to cut the deep transverse intermetatarsal ligament from proximal to distal.
    - Perform osteotomies by placing a full cutting straight 2.0-mm burr on the dorsal, distal metaphyseal aspect of the metatarsal, being sure that the cut is extra-articular, and angling it 45° plantar and proximal to the metatarsal.
    - No fixation is performed on these osteotomies, allowing the distal segments to shift dorsally, increasing the intermetatarsal space.
  - Results:
    - Initial follow-up:

- Postoperative forefoot functional scores are found to have significant improvements when compared with their preoperation reports.
  - At 2- and 7-year follow-up:
    - 25/26 patients report complete relief.
    - This group has continued to have improved functional scores with only 4% presenting with persistent metatarsalgia, whereas the excision group has 44% present with persistent metatarsalgia.
      - Significant finding.

Surgical Complications

Table 1 is a compilation of results from the studies listed in the primary and recurrent treatment options for neuromas. The number of procedures performed for each intervention should be appreciated so that the percent of success is not inflated when comparing.

RECURRENCE

The recurrence rate after a neurectomy ranges from 14% to 21%.[33] For those who present with recurrent symptoms within 12 months of the excision, it may be caused by insufficient resection, whereas if symptoms recur after 12 months from the excision, a stump neuroma could be the cause. When resecting a neuroma, it should be resected to the level of the muscle belly to allow for adequate retraction.[9] A study by Johnson and colleagues[13] looked at 37 resected recurrent neuromas histologically and found 19% to be primary neuromas, 22% stump neuromas, 44% a combination of the two, and 15% pathology not related to neuromas. The persistent pain in most of these patients was then related to the improper resecting by either leaving part of the neuroma intact or failing to resect proximal enough to allow adequate retraction. This emphasizes the proper technique that must be considered when performing a neurectomy on a primary neuroma, which we recommend is to resect at the level of the muscle belly. In the case that recurrence does present in a patient, recommended revisional procedures are as follows.

Treatment

- Neurectomy:
  - Longitudinal plantar incision is the method of choice for revisional neurectomies.
    - Richardson and Dean[6] relates it to the anatomic position of a stump neuroma, stating that it sits more proximal along the common digital nerve compared with a primary neuroma.
    - Johnson and colleagues[13] performed this approach for a neurectomy on 32 of the patients presenting with recurrent symptoms.
      - 66% reported little or no pain at follow-up.
      - Because of these poor results, physicians again seek options to improve recurrent neuroma treatment.
- Nerve transposition:
  - All nerve transposition surgical methods discussed in primary neuroma treatment are used for recurrent neuromas as well.
  - Metatarsal transposition[37]:
    - Methods:
      - Perform a longitudinal plantar approach to access the stump neuroma along with a dorsal incision, medial or lateral to the third metatarsal shaft, depending on which interspace is involved.

Table 1
Success rate and complications of surgical interventions

Surgical Intervention	Long-Term Success (>1 y)	Complications
Decompression (n = 87)	86.2%	5 neurectomies, 3 superficial infections
Dorsal excision (n = 662)	76.7%	50 numbness, 23 MPJ pain, 19 recurrent pain, 13 paresthesia, 10 superficial infections, 2 missed nerves, 1 DVT, 1 CRPS, 1 scar, 1 dehiscence
Plantar excision (n = 265)	88.7%	25 numbness, 19 scars, 7 recurrent pain, 3 paresthesia, 3 superficial infections, 2 missed nerves, 1 cyst, 1 foreign body reaction, 1 hematoma
Dorsal transposition (n = 122)	95.1%	4 neurectomies, 2 numbness, 2 paresthesia
Intermuscular transposition (n = 23)	95.7%	1 infection
Muscle belly transposition[a] (n = 33)	90.9%	2 metatarsalgia, 2 dehiscence, 1 scar
Metatarsal transposition[a] (n = 27)	88.9%	None listed
Nerve graft conduit (n = 9)	77.8%	1 dehiscence
Collagen conduit (n = 54)	92.6%	1 CRPS, 1 persistent pain
Excision with osteotomies (n = 26)	88.5%	1 reoperation, 1 CRPS, 1 progressive hallux valgus, 3 fat pad atrophy, 3 recurrent pain, 3 metatarsalgia

Abbreviations: CRPS, complex regional pain syndrome; DVT, deep vein thrombosis; MPJ, metatarsophalangeal joint.
[a] Recurrent treatment.
Data from Refs.[1,4,5,14,16–18,22,26,31–35,37–39,42,44]

- Use a 5/64-inch drill to make a small hole through the metatarsal shaft.
- Resect the neuroma and pass it through the drill hole.
- Secure the transposed nerve using suture material and a Keith needle.
- Keep the patient nonweightbearing for 3 weeks to prevent the risk of stress fracture.
  - Although this has been a successful procedure, it is not recommended for patients with fat pad atrophy or transfer metatarsalgia.
  - Muscle belly transposition:
    - Transposition into the adductor hallucis brevis[38]:
      - These patients were also found to have tarsal tunnel syndrome diagnosed with a positive Tinel sign and abnormal two-point static touch perception at the hallux and medial heel.
    - Methods:
      - Secure the epineurium of the nerve into the adductor hallucis brevis muscle belly.
      - Tarsal tunnel decompression.
    - 100% of the 17 patients reported good and excellent results.
    - Transposition into the flexor digitorum brevis[14]:
      - Methods:
        - Make a plantar incision with a slight S- or Z-shaped incision.
        - Secure the proximal end of the transected nerve into the flexor digitorum brevis without any tension while the foot is in a dorsiflexed position.

- ○ Keep the patient nonweightbearing for 4 weeks.
  - • 81.3% of the 16 patients reported successful results.
- • Conduits/grafts:
  - ○ Grafts or conduits are used to cover, transpose, or repair a nerve.
  - ○ Collagen conduit[39]:
    - ■ The nerve is resected and the proximal end is placed into a collagen conduit and secured distally and dorsally.
    - ■ 93% of the patients treated with intermetatarsal neuromas are found to be satisfied with their outcomes with a median follow-up of 36 months.
  - ○ Vein conduit[15]:
    - ■ Dorsal transposition of the proximal nerve end is performed and it is suggested to use a vein conduit only when the nerve end is too short to pass dorsally without creating too much tension.
  - ○ Polyglycolic acid conduit[40]:
    - ■ Its structure keeps the nerve inside safe, preventing fibroblast ingrowth and kinking and promoting oxygen diffusion.
    - ■ This study uses conduits to reconnect the proximal and distal nerve ends on the hand, and no complications are found to be directly related to the material itself.
    - ■ 100% of the procedures repairing nerve gaps less than or equal to 4 mm are found to have good results.
  - ○ Nerve allograft conduit[41]:
    - ■ This study treats painful neuromas after amputation.
    - ■ Method:
      - • Use nerve allograft entubated into a porcine submucosa nerve conduit to connect the two ends of the resected and now healthy nerve.
  - ○ Nerve autograft conduit:
    - ■ The study by Bibbo and Rodrigues-Colazzo[41] also suggests that if the damaged nerve is homogeneously sensory, which the second and third common plantar digital nerves are, a healthy segment can be harvested to use as an autograft instead.
    - ■ Ratanshi and colleagues[42] also performed a study using autograft conduits.
      - • Methods:
        - ○ Use a dorsal approach for excision of neuroma.
        - ○ Harvest a segment of the proper plantar digital nerve distal to the excision.
        - ○ Connect the two ends using 9–0 nylon suture under loupe magnification.

DISCUSSION

Proper understanding of neuroma cause and biology aids in providing appropriate care to limit recurrence in neuromas. One must understand that although a primary neuroma is classified as an entrapment syndrome, performing decompression alone may not be a sufficient method of treatment. Although decompression has a good success rate in the study by Barrett and Walsh,[5] Mann and Reynolds[8] found the deep transverse intermetatarsal ligament to repair itself after a decompression, so the issue is only temporarily fixed. The newer, dorsal suspension procedures performed along with ligament decompression show how enhancements have been made based on the understanding of the syndrome.[17,35,39]

Correct diagnosis is another factor when deciding appropriate treatment of metatarsalgia syndrome. A 10.3% of patients in the Johnson and colleagues[13] study was misdiagnosed as a neuroma, which was not acknowledged until the excisional procedure was performed. A similar finding was reported in the study by Haddad and colleagues[43] on crossover toe deformity treatment. Seven patients achieved relief of their forefoot pain from this procedure after dealing with persistent pain to which neurectomies provided little to no relief. This is a challenge because of the similar presentations, so it is important to keep other differentials in mind.

It is also important to weigh the complications and success rates when deciding on an appropriate treatment option. Based on the studies reviewed in this article, the dorsal approach for excision is accompanied with a higher rate of more concerning complications when compared with the plantar approach's mainly scar-related complications.[22,31] Although the comparison of dorsal and plantar approach for excision continues to be the topic of debate, it is important to consider the new, possibly more effective procedures available involving the use of transposition and/or conduits.[14,17,34,35,37–39,42]

Along with the appropriate procedure choice, proper technique may be among the most influential factors when aiming to reduce recurrence. When performing an excision, removing the entire neuroma and resecting proximal enough for sufficient retraction to limit irritation is key. Another suggested technique includes securing nerve transposition procedures with suture, as discussed by Banks and colleagues.[14]

If recurrence does occur, nerve transposition or using a conduit for covering the nerve, transposing it, or repairing it may be more effective than the longitudinal plantar approach for excision. Stump neuromas are commonly found to be adhered to the third metatarsal, skin, joint capsule, and other surrounding structures. This adherence becomes irritated from the constant movement in the plantar foot, which causes pain.[6,34,38] These methods of treatment can prevent the recurrence of adhesions, and ultimately, pain. Although research on using conduits for interdigital neuroma treatment is limited, there have been significant advances for nerve repair documented in nerves with critical functions.[15,40,41]

SUMMARY

Recurrent pain after neuroma surgery is caused by continued extrinsic compression from metatarsal heads or deep transverse intermetatarsal ligament, intrinsic compression from microscopic or macroscopic changes in the nerve, or stump neuroma formation.[42] The reasons for these occurrences have been discussed throughout this article including misunderstanding of cause, misdiagnosis, and improper primary treatment, either by treatment option or technique. Staying cautious of these potential setbacks may reduce recurrent pain associated with neuromas. It is important to be open to patients about these challenges associated with neuromas so that there is a level of understanding when deciding appropriate treatment of primary and revisional care.

DISCLOSURE

The authors have nothing to disclose.

REFERENCES

1. Bennett GL, Graham CE, Mauldin DM. Morton's interdigital neuroma: comprehensive treatment protocol. Foot Ankle Int 1995;16:760–3.

2. Morton T. A peculiar and painful affection of the fourth metatarsal-phalangeal articulation. J Med Sci 1876;167:214.
3. Nissen KI. The etiology of Morton's metatarsalgia. J Bone Joint Surg 1951;33-B: 293–4.
4. Gauthier G. Thomas Morton's disease: a nerve entrapment syndrome. A new surgical technique. Clin Orthop 1979;142:90–2.
5. Barrett SL, Walsh AS. Endoscopic decompression of intermetatarsal nerve entrapment: a retrospective study. J Am Podiatr Med Assoc 2006;96(1):19–23.
6. Richardson DR, Dean EM. The recurrent Morton neuroma: now what? Foot Ankle Clin N Am 2014;19:437–49.
7. Bradley N, Miller WA, Evans JP. Plantar neuroma: analysis of results following surgical excision in 145 patients. South Med J 1976;69:853–4.
8. Mann RA, Reynolds JC. Interdigital neuroma—a critical clinical analysis. Foot Ankle 1983;3:238–43.
9. Di Caprio F, Meringolo R, Eddine MS, et al. Morton's interdigital neuroma of the foot: a literature review. Foot Ankle Surg 2018;24:92–8.
10. Giannini S, Bacchini P, Ceccarelli F, et al. Interdigital neuroma: clinical examination and histopathologic results in 63 cases treated with excision. Foot Ankle Int 2004;25:79–84.
11. Giakoumis M, Ryan J, Jani J. Histologic evaluation of intermetatarsal Morton's neuroma. J Am Poidatr Med Assoc 2013;103(3):218–22.
12. Morscher E, Urlich J, Dick W. Morton's intermetatarsal neuroma: morphology and histological substrate. Foot Ankle 2000;21(7):558–62.
13. Johnson JE, Johnson KA, Unni KK. Persistent pain after excision of an interdigital neuroma: results of reoperation. J Bone Joint Surg 1988;70A:651–7.
14. Banks AS, Vito GR, Giorgini TL. Recurrent intermetatarsal neuroma: a follow-up study. J Am Podiatr Med Assoc 1996;86(7):299–306.
15. Wagner E, Ortiz C. The painful neuroma and the use of conduits. Foot Ankle Clin 2011;16:295–304.
16. Coughlin MJ, Schenck RC, Shurnas PJ, et al. Concurrent interdigital neuroma and MTP joint instability: long-term results of treatment. Foot Ankle Int 2002; 23(11):1018–25.
17. Vito GR, Talarico LM. A modified technique for Morton's neuroma: decompression with relocation. J Am Podiatr Med Assoc 2003;93(3):190–4.
18. Bauer T, Gaumetou E, Klouche S, et al. Metatarsalgia and Morton's disease: comparison of outcomes between open procedure and neurectomy versus percutaneous metatarsal osteotomies and ligament release with a minimum of 2 years of follow-up. J Foot Ankle Surg 2015;54:373–7.
19. Guiloff RJ, Scadding JW, Klenerman L. Morton's metatarsalgia: clinical, electrophysiological and histological observations. J Bone Joint Surg 1984;66-B(4): 586–91.
20. Dellon AL, Mackinnon SE. Treatment of the painful neuroma by neuroma resection and muscle implantation. Plast Reconstr Surg 1986;77(3):427–36.
21. Mulder JD. The causative mechanism in Morton's metatarsalgia. J Bone Joint Surg 1951;33-B(1):94–5.
22. Akermark C, Crone H, Skoog A, et al. A prospective randomized controlled trial of plantar versus dorsal incisions for operative treatment of primary Morton's neuroma. Foot Ankle Int 2013;34(9):1198–204.
23. Fazal MA, Khan I, Thomas C. Ultrasonography and magnetic resonance imaging in the diagnosis of Morton's neuroma. J Am Podiatr Med Assoc 2012;102(3): 184–6.

24. Ata AM, Onat SS, Ozcakar L. Ultrasound-guided diagnosis and treatment of Morton's neuroma. Pain Physician 2016;19-E:355–7.
25. Read JW, Noakes JB, Kerr D, et al. Morton's metatarsalgia: sonographic findings and correlated histopathology. Foot Ankle 1999;20(3):153–61.
26. Greenfield J, Rea J, Ilfield F. Morton's interdigital neuroma: indications for treatment by local injections versus surgery. Clin Orthop Relat Res 1984;185:142–4.
27. Musson RE, Sawhney JS, Lamb L, et al. Ultrasound guided alcohol ablation of Morton's neuroma. Foot Ankle Int 2012;33(3):196–201.
28. Hughes RJ, Ali K, Jones H, et al. Treatment of Morton's neuroma with alcohol injection under sonographic guidance: follow-up of 101 cases. AJR Am J Roentgenol 2007;188:1535–9.
29. Gurdezi S, White T, Ramesh P. Alcohol injection for Morton's neuroma: a five-year follow-up. Foot Ankle Int 2013;34(8):1064–7.
30. Post MD, Maccio JR. Mechanical diagnosis and therapy and Morton's neuroma: a case-series. J Man ManipTher 2019. https://doi.org/10.1080/10669817.2019.1611044.
31. Akermark C, Crone H, Saartok T, et al. Plantar versus dorsal incisions in the treatment of primary intermetatarsal Morton's neuroma. Foot Ankle Int 2008;29:136–41.
32. Nery C, Raduan F, Del Buono A, et al. Plantar approach for excision of a Morton neuroma: a long-term follow-up study. J Bone Joint Surg Am 2012;94(7):654–8.
33. Faraj AA, Hosur A. The outcome after using two different approaches for excision of Morton's neuroma. Chin Med J 2010;123(16):2195–8.
34. Colgrove RC, Huang EY, Barth AH, et al. Interdigital neuroma: intermuscular neuroma transposition compared with resection. Foot Ankle Int 2000;21(3):206–11.
35. Song JH, Kang C, Hwang DS, et al. Dorsal suspension for Morton's neuroma: a comparison with neurectomy. Foot Ankle Surg 2019;25(6):748–54.
36. Koch H, Herbert TJ, Kleinert R, et al. Influence of nerve stump transplantation into a vein on neuroma formation. Ann Plast Surg 2003;50(4):354–60.
37. Nelms BA, Bishop JO, Tullos HS. Surgical treatment of recurrent Morton's neuroma. Orthop J 1984;7(2):1708–11.
38. Wolfort SF, Dellon AL. Treatment of recurrent neuroma of the interdigital nerve by implantation of the proximal nerve into muscle in the arch of the foot. J Foot Ankle Surg 2001;40(6):404–10.
39. Gould JS, Naranje SM, McGwin G, et al. Use of collagen conduits in management of painful neuromas of the foot and ankle. Foot Ankle Int 2013;34(7):932–40.
40. Weber RA, Breidenbach WC, Brown RE, et al. A randomized prospective study of polyglycolic acid conduits for digital nerve reconstruction in humans. Plast Reconstr Surg 2000;106:1036–45.
41. Bibbo C, Rodrigues-Colazzo E. Nerve transfer with entubated nerve allograft transfers to treat recalcitrant lower extremity neuromas. J Foot Ankle Surg 2017;56:82–6.
42. Ratanshi I, Hayakawa TEJ, Giuffre JL. Excision with interpositional nerve grafting: an alternative technique for the treatment of Morton neuroma. Ann Plast Surg 2016;76:428–33.
43. Haddad SL, Sabbagh RC, Resch S, et al. Results of flexor-to-extensor and extensor brevis tendon transfer for correction of the crossover second toe deformity. Foot Ankle Int 1999;20(12):781–8.
44. Womack JW, Richardson DR, Murphy GA, et al. Long-term evaluation of interdigital neuroma treated by surgical excision. Foot Ankle Int 2008;29(6):574–7.

Osteochondral Lesions of the Talar Dome

Mitchell J. Thompson, DPM[a],*, Thomas S. Roukis, DPM, PhD[b]

KEYWORDS

- Osteochondral talar dome lesion • Cystic lesion • Microfracture • Bulk talar allograft

KEY POINTS

- When an osteochondral lesion of the talar dome (OCLT) is suspected, a magnetic resonance image has higher sensitivity but a computed tomographic scan has higher specificity in terms of size and extent of the osseous destruction.
- Nonsurgical treatment should be considered first in OCLT cases, even though studies show low success rates.
- The size and location of the lesion greatly dictate the preferred surgical procedure.

INTRODUCTION

Osteochondral lesion of the talar dome (OCLT) is a term that encompasses any injury to the articulating cartilage of the talus. The term OCLT was first described in 1887 by Konig and 35 years later, in 1922, another common name, *osteochondritis dissecans of the talar dome*, was coined by Kappis.[1] Ever since these descriptions, OCTLs have been an increasing diagnosis for ankle pain. The exact incidence is indeterminate simply because not all are symptomatic, and many are undetected for this reason. The best incidence estimate is due to a study by Orr and colleagues,[2] in 2011, a 10-year study looking at military personnel, which estimated the incidence to be 27 per 100,000.

The cause of OCTLs has been an area of major debate for many years. Trauma repeatedly has been found to be the main etiology of these lesions; this can be from an isolated single event or from years of repetitive microtrauma.[3] Even though trauma has been linked to the main cause of OCLTs, idiopathic OCLTs do occur. Studies have shown that symptomatic OCLTs are associated with 6.5% of all ankle sprains and up to 50% of all ankle sprains and acute ankle fractures can lead to an OCLT.[3,4]

[a] Gundersen Medical Foundation, Gundersen Health System, 1900 South Avenue, La Crosse, WI 54601, USA; [b] Orthopaedic Center, Gundersen Health System, 1900 South Avenue, La Crosse, WI 54601, USA
* Corresponding author. Mail Stop CO3-006A, 1900 South Avenue, La Crosse, WI 54601.
E-mail address: mjthomps@gundersenhealth.org

Clin Podiatr Med Surg 37 (2020) 533–551
https://doi.org/10.1016/j.cpm.2020.02.002
0891-8422/20/© 2020 Elsevier Inc. All rights reserved.

The typical clinic presentation can be either acute or chronic. Patients likely have deep ankle pain that they can relate to some type of injury or inciting event. Inciting events may be things, such as increase in weight-bearing activity, more ballistic type of activity, or anything that increases pressures in an axial load to the ankle joint. The most common time patients experience this type of pain is either during the activity or after. Stiffness and swelling are other common symptoms that occur with OCLTs but rarely is range of motion limited.

Traditional thinking describes 2 predominant areas where OCLTs typically are found anterior lateral and posterior medial. It has been suggested that a majority of the anterior lateral lesions do have a traumatic etiology.[5] Raikin and colleagues[6] challenged this concept and evaluated 424 patients using magnetic resonance imaging (MRI) and an anatomic grid to look at locations of OCLTs. They found the most common areas of lesions were center-medial and center-lateral at 53.0% and 25.7%, respectively.[7] Anterior lateral lesions occur when the ankle is forcibly dorsiflexed and inverted at the same time, thus creating an interaction between the anterior lateral talar dome and the fibula. The posterior medial lesions, although they may be traumatic, also have a higher likelihood of being idiopathic. The posterior medial lesion is caused by plantarflexion and inversion of the ankle joint.[8] Upon plantarflexion and inversion of the ankle, the posterior medial talar dome makes contact with the tibial plafond, causing injury.

It is important to distinguish or exclude all other possible pathologies that could exist in or around the ankle joint itself, and typically weight-bearing radiographs of the ankle is first-line imaging. Anterior-posterior, mortise, and lateral views of the ankle are the views needed at minimum; others may be added depending on surgeon preference. One such special view is a mortise view of the ankle while the ankle also is in plantarflexion. Verhagen and colleagues[9] published a comparison study utilizing this mortise view with the heels on a 4-cm lift. This view diagnosed posterior talar dome lesions most accurately and proved superior to helical computed tomography (CT) for posterior lesions. Acute OCLTs, unless quite large, often are difficult to appreciate on radiographs. Chronic OCLTs can be appreciated by radiolucency and possible cartilage depression in severe cases. A radiograph image rarely is sensitive enough to diagnose and fully evaluate an OCLT; thus, advanced imaging is indicated.

MRI often is considered the imaging modality of choice for a suspected OCLT. It has been shown that an MRI can detect up to 50% of OCLTs that otherwise would be missed on plain film radiographs.[10] Obtaining MRI slices in the sagittal, frontal, and axial planes are vital for proper measurement of the exact size of the lesion. At minimum, these views all should be obtained in T1-weighted and T2-weighted images. On T1 fat-enhancing imaging, sclerosis of the OCLT shows up as a low signal intensity. The T2 image shows if there is any fluid collection around the osteochondral lesion of the talus (OCLT) or, in some cases, separation of the OCLT from the talar body.[11] Any bone marrow edema shows up as a hypertense signal within the talar dome on a T2 image and low signal intensity on a T1. Cystic changes within the talus also may be observed in a talar body susceptible to an OCLT. The contents within the cysts determine the signal intensity on the MRIs.[12] Another advantage of MRI with an OCLT is that it allows for inspection of the surrounding ankle ligaments and tendons for other associated pathology. In the authors' opinion, MRI is the modality of choice for the most efficacious diagnostic tool to diagnose an OCLT, although once an OCLT is diagnosed and the surrounding structures assessed, a CT scan is best for surgical planning.

A CT scan is beneficial in determining the entire extent of the OCLT due to its ability to better differentiate viable from nonviable bone. Therefore, a CT may provide a more accurate measurements of the size. At CT scan also ishelpful in evaluating subchondral or talar cysts that may be present within the bone. A CT scan is not be able to determine if there is a loose body within the OCLT nor does it allow for assessment of the surrounding soft tissue. Intra-articular contrast can be used in conjunction with a CT scan. Intra-articular contrast may help visualize loose bodies better by showing the free space under the loose body and indicating cystic lesions to better assess the extent of subchondral cysts.

Although becoming less common with the increased sensitivity and specificity of the modalities discussed previously, bone scan remains a viable option for detection of an OTL. Studies have shown a bone scan, specifically technetium 99m, to detect up to 99% of OCLTs.[9] Bone scintigraphy is shown to have a 94% sensitivity to OTLs when missed on radiographs.[13]

Single-photon emission CT (SPECT) is a newer type of scan that is not available at many institutions but warrants mentioning. SPECT combines imaging techniques from both a bone scan and CT to provide more accurate and specific images. SPECT has been shown to provide more accurate images to the exact size of the lesion and be more sensitive to changes in the OCLT compared with an MRI.[14]

CLASSIFICATIONS

The most common classification system regarding OCLTs was described in 1959 by Berndt and Harty[15] (**Table 1**). This classification is widely used to stage the severity of the lesion in terms of the cartilage being intact and state of the underlying subchondral bone. This classification is based solely on radiographic findings.

The original Berndt and Harty classification have been adapted and modified throughout the years as imaging modalities have become more advanced. In 1991, Dipaola and colleagues[16] adapted the original Berndt and Harty classification but added the MRI findings associated with each of the 4 stages. Soon after, in 1999, Hepple and colleagues[17] developed a similar OCLT classification utilizing MRI findings but separated stage 2 into 2a, cartilage with underlying fracture and bone marrow edema, and 2b, cartilage with underlying fracture without bone marrow edema. They also

Table 1 Berndt and Harty classification	
Stage	**Description of Lesion**
I	Compression/depression of the subchondral bone of the talus
II	Partial detachment of the osteochondral fragment
III	Complete detachment of the osteochondral fragment, but the fragment is nondisplaced
IV	Complete detachment of the osteochondral fragment with the fragment displaced

Data from Meftah M, Katchis SD, Scharf, SC, et al. SPECT/CT in the management of osteochondral lesions of the talus. Foot & Ankle International. 2011;32(3):233-238.

added a stage 5 to include subchondral cyst formation in the setting of an OTL. Ferkel and colleagues[18] developed an OTL classification based on CT findings in 1994. This classification focused on osseous pathology, including cystic changes in its first 2 stages. All classification systems aim to determine the severity of the lesion and give insight into the damage done to the chondral and subchondral bone. These classifications are helpful because, as discussed later, the stage of the lesion may indicate or contraindicate certain treatment options.

CONSERVATIVE TREATMENTS

After an OCLT is confirmed, a wide array of treatment options exists (**Fig. 1**), with nonsurgical treatments typically used for a period of 6 weeks to 6 months prior to pursuing surgical options. The goal of nonsurgical treatment is to decrease edema around the damaged lesion and immobilize the area enough to allow the subchondral bone lesion to repair itself and cartilage to scar back down to the subchondral bone.[19] Nonsurgical treatments consist of either minimizing weight-bearing activity or making patients completely non–weight bearing. In either case, the ankle frequently is kept at a 90° angle in a cast or a removable boot. Supportive measures typically also are used, such as nonsteroidal anti-inflammatory drugs, cryotherapy, elevation, compression, and physical therapy treatment/modalities. Nonoperative treatment has been shown successful up to 45% of the time, allowing patients to return to their prior activities.[20,21] After a period of 6 weeks to 8 weeks of nonsurgical treatment, patients are able to determine if any marked progress is being made; if symptoms have stayed the same or worsened during this time period, surgical options should begin to be discussed.

SURGICAL TREATMENT

When OCLTs are severe enough or conservative treatments fail, surgery often is undertaken, although which surgical treatment to pursue is not always clear. Multiple

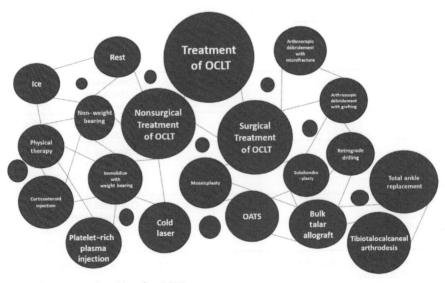

Fig. 1. Treatment algorithm for OCLT.

surgical options exist, and many are dependent on the stage, location, and size of the lesion (see **Fig. 1; Table 2**). Smaller lesions that fall into the stage 2 to stage 4 areas usually can be treated through arthroscopic means. Larger lesions that are displaced and detached may need a more open or minimal incisional approach. Surgical treatment typically is performed with 1 of 3 different techniques: (1) débridement, (2) internal fixation, or (3) variation of grafting measures.

ARTHROSCOPY WITH MICROFRACTURING

Access to the ankle joint on smaller lesions often can be performed through arthroscopic techniques. This allows minimal incisions to be utilized, decreasing risk for postoperative complications. Arthroscopic treatment of OCLTs with microfracturing is recommended for lesions smaller than 2 cm^2.[22] The microfracture technique is utilized to stimulate the underlying bone marrow to create fibrocartilage.[23] Portal placement is surgeon preference, but in most cases lesions can be assessed through standard anterior portals. Once the ankle joint is properly visualized, the lesion is identified. A blunt probe then is inserted through the instrument portal to identify and assess the OCLT, deciphering the exact size of the lesion and the demarcation of where the cartilage is still attached to underlying bone. A pituitary rongeur or any type of grasper then can be used to remove the loose cartilage and any debris that

Table 2
Osteochondral lesion of the talar dome surgical options

Surgical Treatment	Stage	Size	Graft/Biologics	Surgical Approach	Average Increase in AOFAS Score
Arthroscopy with microfracture	II, IV	<1.5 cm^2	None	Arthroscopic	25.1[24]
Arthroscopy with bone graft	II–IV	<1.5 cm^2	Auto, Allograft, Biologics	Arthroscopic	36[35]
Subchondroplasty	I, II	<1.5 cm^2	Biologics	Minimally invasive/ arthroscopic	22.5[35]
Retrograde drilling	I, II	<1.5 cm^2	None	Minimally invasive /arthroscopic	34[36]
Osteochondral autograft transfer system	III–IV	1.5-3 cm^2	Autograft	Arthroscopic or open	28[37]
Mosaicplasty	III–IV	1.5–3 cm^2	Autograft	Arthroscopic or open	39[38]
Bulk talar allograft	V	>1.5 cm^2	Autograft	Open malleolar osteotomy	36[39]
TAR	Revision	>3 cm^2	None	Open anterior	—
TTC	Revision	>3 cm^2	Auto/allograft	Open lateral vascularized fibular onlay graft	—

Data from Refs.[24,35,35–39]

is present. OCLT often is described as crater-like, meaning there is a step-off from the healthy cartilage to the subchondral bone. An arthroscopic burr can be used to burr down the step offs into a more gradually slope. Next, the microfracturing can occur; this typically is done best with a microfracture awl. The microfracture technique should include penetrating through the subchondral plate to allow pluripotent stem cells to fill the OTL, creating a fibrocartilaginous covering of the defect. This depth typically 2 is mm but often can be visualized by appearance of fat bubbles after penetrating through the plate. These microfractures also should be spaced 3 mm to 4 mm apart.[24] Once the lesion has been completely microfractured, the portals are closed, and typical postoperative protocol is non–weight bearing in a splint or ankle immobilization boot for 6 weeks, with gradual return to activity afterward.

In 2012, Donnenwerth and Roukis[25] undertook a systematic review evaluating 29 total articles, of which 7 met inclusion criteria, on patient outcomes after arthroscopic débridement with microfracturing. This study encompassed 295 total patients and 299 ankles. All patients had undergone arthroscopic debridement with microfracture and, at a mean follow-up of 54 months, the investigators determined an average increase in the American Orthopaedic Foot and Ankle Society (AOFAS) score of 25.1 points. The investigators stated this correlated to a good or excellent outcome in 80% of the ankles after surgery. The most common complication found was superficial peroneal nerve injury.[25]

ARTHROSCOPY WITH BONE GRAFT

There is a strong correlation of cystic changes within the talus when an OCLT is presenting. Some studies suggest these cystic changes can be present up to 25% of the time.[26] Often these OCLTs can be approached in a manner similar to that described previously, with the exception of the need to fill the cystic lesion to provide a foundation for the OCLT to repair itself after débridement. It has been described that an OCLT with loose cartilage can have a valve-like effect, allowing fluid from the ankle to enter under the cartilage but not escape, and the continuation of this process is what creates the cystic lesion.[27] In the investigators' experience, lesions on the shoulder of the talus are difficult to treat with bone graft and osteobiologics alone and made even more difficult arthroscopically; the authors advocate for an open approach, as explained later, for shoulder lesions. Once a decision is made to approach the lesion arthroscopically, the standard anterior portals can be made for an anterior-lateral lesion. It is surgeon preference if a posterior approach provides best access to any posterior medial lesions. Once identified, the lesion is débrided with surgeon's choice of arthroscopic instruments. It is important to thoroughly débride the cystic lesion. It also is good technique to drill the lesion as well; this can be done with Kirschner wires or a microfracture awl. Next, a cannulated device is placed through the instrument portal, which delivers the bone graft directly into the prepared cystic lesion, limiting excess spill into the ankle joint. After the cyst is filled, the graft is then impacted and this process is continued until the void is tightly packed with bone graft. The postoperative protocol is similar to that described previously, with the patient in a posterior splint and immobilized with non–weight bearing for a minimum of 6 weeks.

SUBCHONDROPLASTY/RETROGRADE DRILLING

Subchondroplasty treatment has specific indications because this is a treatment to repair the underlying subchondral bone, although the authors believe it warrants discussion. A subchondroplasty is done by retrograde filling a subchondral bone defect with osteobiologics or some type of bone matrix with primarily calcium phosphate base.[28] In order for this process to be successful, there must be intact overlying cartilage or intact bone so that the contents cannot leak out into the ankle joint. This can be done in conjunction with an arthroscopic débridement. The introduction of the osteobiologic can be done directly through the OCLT or from a retrograde-type fashion. The goal of this procedure is to allow solidification of the underlying bone and provide a solid base, which limit the potential breakdown of the overlying cartilage.

Retrograde drilling of the underlying lesions also is discussed because the principals are similar. This technique is used under similar indications in which the overlying cartilage is in good repair. The goal of this procedure is to stimulate the subchondral bone using the same principals as micrfracturing.

OSTEOCHONDRAL AUTOGRAFT TRANSFER SYSTEM/MOSAICPLASTY

Lesions larger than 1.5 cm^2 are have a lower success rate when treated purely through microfracture means, and likely some sort of open grafting is utilized. In 2004, Hangody and colleagues[29] described an autologous osteochondral mosaicplasty technique. This technique involves removing small cylindrical subchondral grafts from the non–weight-bearing part of the femoral condyle and transferring them down to the talar defect. A cylindrical recipient defect is made overlying the OTL and the graft then is transferred and impacted; no fixation is necessary. The aim of this is to replace the damaged hyaline cartilage with new hyaline cartilage. Although this procedure can be done arthroscopically, the investigators advocate for a miniarthrotomy. In their initial study on this procedure Hangody and colleagues[29] showed a 94% good to excellent result in the patients undergoing a mosaicplasty for an OCLT.

MEDIAL MALLEOLAR OSTEOTOMY WITH BULK TALAR ALLOGRAFT

Larger OCLTs greater than 1.5 cm^2 with underlying cystic lesions involving the shoulder of the talar dome often are difficult to treat with the treatments discussed previously.[30] Most of the prior studies, which aimed to look at the treatments of these larger lesions, used structural bulk talar allograft treatment algorithm. The bulk talar allograft not only allows the surgeon to replace large voids within the talar dome but also provides a structural integrity to the allograft that allows for repair of OCLTs that involve the shoulder of the talus.

The exact size of the lesion is estimated through advanced imaging in the form of a CT scan. A donor talus then can be ordered not only to ensure ability to obtain a proper-sized graft but also to match gender and age of the donor graft with the surgical patient.

The OCLT can be accessed in multiple different ways and can be performed per surgeon preference. The authors' preference is to perform a medial or lateral malleolar osteotomy to gain access to the lesions. In the authors' experience, a medial talar shoulder lesion has been most prevalent and the authors will continue with this surgical technique. An oblique cut is made from proximal medial into the ankle joint, ensuring the distal lateral exit point allows complete access to the OCLT. Just before exiting into the ankle joint with the sagittal saw, the saw is removed and an osteotome is inserted to complete and pry open the osteotomy to create an irregular/jagged fracture through the remaining osteotomy, including the subchondral bone and cartilage. This unique fracture pattern allows for only 1 correct reduction of the osteotomy at the completion of the procedure. Before reflecting down the medial malleolus, while the medial malleolus is properly in place, 2 Kirschner wires may be placed and then backed out to ensure proper guide hole placement for the fixation screws at the end. The medial malleolus now is reflected distally to keep the deltoid ligament attachments intact. The OCLT is identified and a proper border is drawn to ensure complete removal of the entire OCLT and cyst. The OCLT then is resected using a sagittal saw, creating a rectangular shaped void. Multiple measurements are taken of the void in all dimensions.

On a back table, the frozen allograft is soaking in a mixture of sterile saline impregnated with gentamycin (Fresenius Kabi USA, Lake Zurich, Illinois). The authors use frozen talar allografts because these are more readily available and less expensive; to the authors' knowledge, there is no discernible difference between autograft and allograft in osseous incorporation. The allograft is placed on a cutting board and 1 assistant secures the graft with a sharp towel clamp to avoid any movement during cutting or the graft slipping off of the table. Using the measurements obtained and on the proper talar shoulder, the graft is drawn out and a sagittal saw is used to cut out the graft. A pearl to this technique is to place a threaded Kirschner wire into the graft piece that is being cut out in the precise location a screw would go into. This allows handling and stabilizing the graft as well as facilitating placement and stabilization of the graft into the donor site. Once the graft is cut, there are multiple trips back to the operating table to assess fit of the graft. The graft should fit tightly within the donor site and without step-off on the articulating surface. The graft then is fixated with headless screws. The ankle joint is irrigated thoroughly, and then medial malleolar osteotomy is reduced and fixated properly.

Orr and colleagues,[31] in 2016, performed a retrospective study looking at fresh bulk talar allograft in highly active individuals. The study consisted of 8 procedures performed from 2010 to 2013. All procedures were performed in a fashion similar to that described previously. The average size of the defect after excision was 2.25 cm³. All 8 patients went on to heal their bulk talar allografts. At final follow-up of 28.5 months, all patients fully healed their bulk talar allografts, with an average increase in AOFAS score of 47% and a decrease in visual analog scale (VAS) score of 35%.[31] In a systematic review in 2017 looking at 91 bulk talar allografts for OCLTs, VanTienderen and colleagues[32] found an average of a 40% increase in AOFAS scores and a 62% decrease in overall VAS pain scores.

TOTAL ANKLE REPLACEMENT/TIBIOTALOCALCANEAL ARTHRODESIS

Total ankle replacement (TAR) and tibiotalocalcaneal arthrodesis (TTC) procedures are reserved for severe nonsalvageable OCLTs or as revision treatments after failed prior procedures. Patient factors and goals play a large role in determining which treatment to pursue. Ankle joints with moderate to severe arthrosis should be considered for TAR or TTC, because the procedures, discussed previously, do not address the concomitant arthrosis.[33] A CT scan to assess the OCLT also gives insight to remaining viable talus, which is key for surgical planning. A TAR is considered if the OCLT is able to be excised while maintaining enough talus to perform a TAR, along with the other indications for TAR, not discussed. If the talus is nonsalvageable, then discussions of a TTC with bulk femoral head allografting may need to be considered.

Multiple primary and revision TAR systems are now available, which increase the indications for TAR in the setting of a débrided talus. The talus should be structurally sound to receive the talar component of the TAR. There are indications in which a staged procedure to fill subchondral cysts can be performed with plans to implant a TAR later, although this is outside the confines of this article. Another consideration is any varus or valgus imbalances with the ankle joint that may have contributed to the OCLT, which should be addressed at the time of the TAR to provide a rectus ankle joint.

A TTC arthrodesis is a viable and predictable surgery when the talus is nonsalvageable due to large cystic OCLTs, failed prior surgeries, or severe arthrosis in the setting of an OCLT. The authors propose a vascularized fibular onlay graft approach.[34] A fenestrated bulk femoral head allograft is used to fill the void left after débridement of all nonviable talus, although a bulk talar body allograft also can be used. A study in 2018 by Rogero and colleagues[35] looked at 22 cases of TTC arthrodesis with bulk femoral head allograft and found 82% radiographically stable at 39.7 months. The study also stated 73.3% of patients had continued satisfaction with their surgery at 57.1 months.

CASE 1

A 15-year-old girl with an unremarkable past medical history had a 2-year history of ongoing left ankle pain and was referred from an outside provider. The patient was very active in sports and recalled no inciting trauma but did relate to repeatedly twisting her ankle during her activities. The patient did relate to increased pain with plantar flexion and going down stairs. Initial radiographs exhibited findings for a possible OCLT; thus, an MRI without contrast was ordered, which did show an OCLT on the posterior medial aspect of the talar dome (**Figs. 2** and **3**).

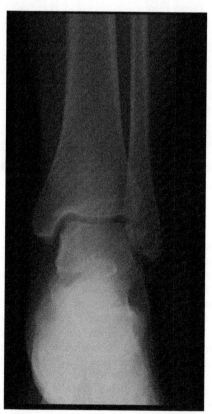

Fig. 2. Anterior-posterior radiographic image of the right ankle, showing a medial shoulder OCLT.

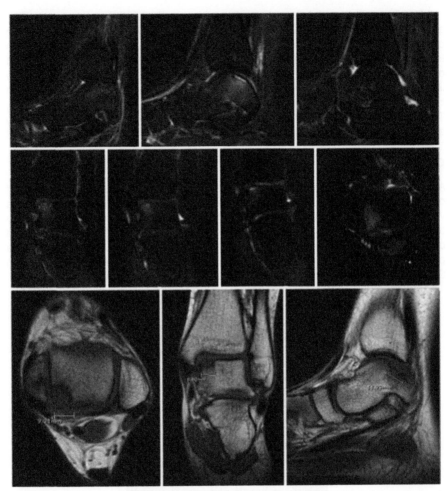

Fig. 3. T2 (*top*) and T1 (*bottom*) MRI, indicating a posterior medial OCLT involving the shoulder of the talus.

The patient had failed appropriate nonsurgical treatments; thus, the patient was consented for arthroscopic débridement of the OCLT with microfracturing of the lesion. The lesion was accessed via standard anterior medial and anterior lateral arthroscopic portals. The lesion was properly identified and débrided (**Fig. 4**A,B). Microfracturing was performed utilizing a microfracture awl (**Fig. 4**C,D). The patient was splinted with the ankle at 90° and made non–weight bearing. The patient was placed in a controlled ankle motion boot at 2 weeks and kept non–weight bearing but allowed to perform range-of-motion exercises and then transition to weight bearing in a boot at 4 weeks. The patient was back to her sports activities without restrictions at 12 weeks.

Unfortunately, the patient was seen back at the 7-month mark with increased left ankle pain. The patient had stated her symptoms were back, reappearing shortly after returning to her aggressive volleyball and swimming activities, and progressively worsened. The patient again presented at an outside institution first, where an MRI

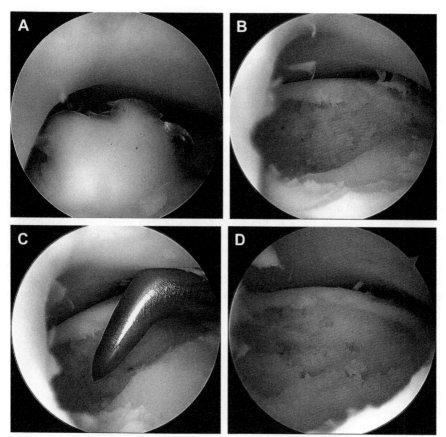

Fig. 4. (*A*) Arthroscopic intraoperative image of the loose OCLT. (*B*) Arthroscopic intraoperative image with the defect noted on the talar dome after removal of loose OCLT. (*C*) Arthroscopic intraoperative image of the microfracturing awl, overlying the OCLT, with gold tip representing 2 mm of depth. (*D*) Arthroscopic intraoperative image of the OCLT lesion after microfracturing of lesion has been completed.

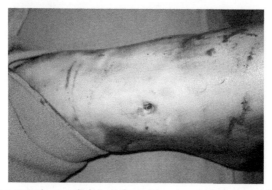

Fig. 5. Nonhealing anterior medial portal probing to ankle joint with MSSA infection 2 months after the second arthroscopic débridement.

was ordered, showing no new OCLT or cystic changes within the talus. The patient was given an ankle brace for symptom management prior to being seen by the senior author (T. Roukis). The patient then presented to the senior author and was enrolled in a physical therapy course while refraining from ballistic-type activities. The patient showed no improvement after 6 weeks of physical therapy. A corticosteroid injection was then given to the ankle with both diagnostic and therapeutic potentials. In office after the injection, yhe patient ambulated pain-free, indicating an intra-articular pathologic process. The effects of the corticosteroid injection had worn off at the 6-week mark and discussion was had for a repeat MRI. MRI showed progressive filling of the old OCLT with no new pathologic processes seen. The patient returned for another corticosteroid injection approximately 5 months lateral prior to her fall sporting activities and then underwent a repeat arthroscopic synovectomy after her sporting season. The patient again had an uneventful recovery from this surgery until the 2-month mark, when she developed a wound with inflammation to the medial portal site that did appear to track to the ankle joint. Cultures were taken indicating a methicillin-sensitive *Staphylococcus aureus* (MSSA) septic joint (**Fig. 5**). The patient was placed on 6 weeks of oral antibiotics per the infectious disease team. The patient was able to heal her wound but approximately 10 days after completing her antibiotics course her ankle became painful and swollen (**Fig. 6**). The patient had a repeated arthroscopic irrigation and drainage of the ankle joint at this time with admission to

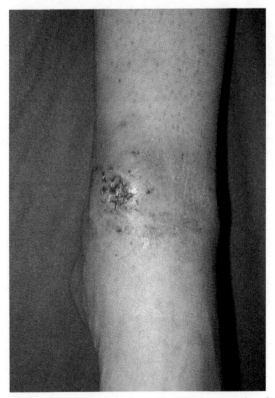

Fig. 6. Anterior medial portal 10 days after completing the 6 weeks of antibiotics for an MSSA septic joint.

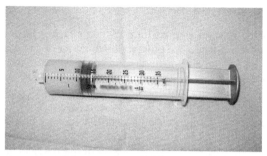

Fig. 7. A 35-mL syringe containing purulent fluid evacuated from the ankle joint after arthroscopic débridement.

the hospital for intravenous antibiotics with peripherally inserted central catheter line placement for 4 weeks of antibiotic infusions followed by 4 weeks of oral antibiotics. Significant purulence was encountered up entry into the ankle joint (**Fig. 7**). Hemorrhagic synovitis and hemarthrosis along with unhealthy appearing fibrocartilage overlying the previous OCLT area was noted and débrided (**Fig. 8**).

The patient was able to heal her skin incisions and remained infection-free after her antibiotic course. She continued with consistent pain to the left ankle but reportedly less than prior to her surgeries, although over time her symptoms to her left ankle progressed, limiting her ability to perform her sporting activities or perform jobs that required weight-bearing activities. Status post 5 years from her initial surgery and 7 years from symptoms developing, the patient had continued pain to her left ankle and was lost to follow-up after seeking a second opinion on options to treat her left ankle. This case demonstrates the potential risks of a routine procedure and potential complications that could lead to more invasive-type procedures, as demonstrated in case 2.

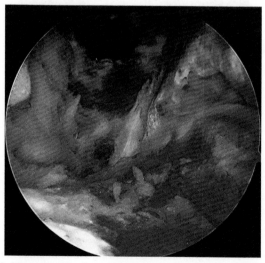

Fig. 8. Arthroscopic intraoperative image showing hemarthrosis of the prior OCLT.

CASE 2

A 38-year-old healthy woman who performed manual labor for a living sustained a right ankle injury while working. The patient could not recall the exact mechanism in which she injured her ankle. Her pain was managed with ice and over-the-counter nonsteroidal anti-inflammatory drugs; thus, the patient did not seek medical care. Due to ongoing symptoms, the patient was seen at an outside institution approximately 3 months after her injury. Radiographs were taken, showing radiolucency of the posterior medial talar dome consistent with osteochondritis dissecans (**Fig. 9**). An MRI without contrast subsequently was ordered to better assess the lesion, demonstrating a 9-mm × 13-mm × 6-mm lesion of the medial talar dome (**Fig. 10**). Due to the size of the lesion, the patient was referred to the authors' institution for discussion on surgical management. The patient was instructed to use an ankle brace and limit ballistic-type activities in the meantime. The patient presented for consultation at the authors' institution approximately 4 months after the initial injury. The patient had continued aching pain to the right ankle joint but discontinued use of the brace and continued to perform manual labor. The patient performed 1 month of nonsurgical treatment, consisting of protected weight bearing in a brace, rest, icing, and compression therapies. She returned after this month with continued discomfort, and a corticosteroid injection was administered to assist with symptom relief. The

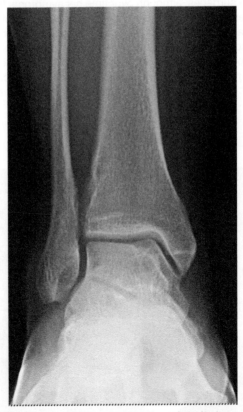

Fig. 9. Anterior-posterior radiographic image showing subtle findings suggestive of OCLT of the medial talar dome.

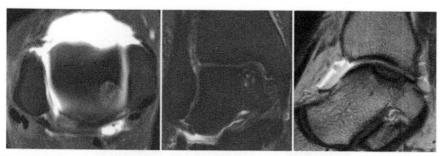

Fig. 10. T1 (*last image*) and T2 (*first two images*) MRI, showing posterior medial OCLT.

corticosteroid injection provided only 2 days to 3 days of symptom relief and the patient presented 1 month later with unchanged symptoms. At this time, a formal custom brace in form of an ankle foot orthosis was recommended and the patient moved forward with custom bracing. The patient received the brace and returned to the clinic approximately 6 months later (1.5 years from initial injury) with continued right ankle pain and swelling. At this time, a CT scan was ordered to assess the lesion and surrounding bone. The CT scan without contrast showed a significant osteochondral

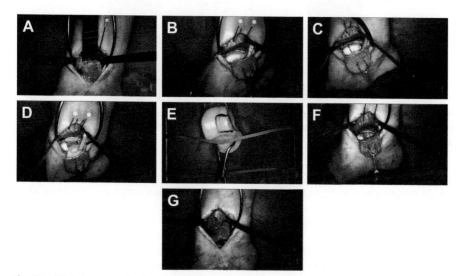

Fig. 11. (*A*) Intraoperative image showing completion of the medial malleolar osteotomy with an osteotome to create an irregular completion of the osteotomy for proper reduction. (*B*) Intraoperative image showing reflection of the medial malleolus inferior about the deltoid ligament to expose the medial shoulder of the talus. (*C*) Intraoperative image showing outline of the OCLT with solid osteochondral margins; outline is done in a rectangular fashion to provide a technically less difficult cut for the allograft. (*D*) Intraoperative image showing defect in talus after removal of the OCLT. (*E*) Intraoperative image indicating securement of the frozen allograft tendon with rubber bands and pointed reduction clamps. Note the rectangular outline of defect on the medial shoulder of the allograft talus. (*F*) Intraoperative image showing allograft properly seated in place and fixated with headless compression screws placed medial to lateral. (*G*) Intraoperative image showing reduction and fixation of the medial malleolar osteotomy with 2 screws running distal to proximal and 2 screws traversing medial to lateral across the osteotomy.

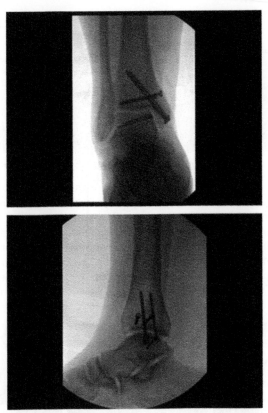

Fig. 12. Anterior-posterior (*top*) and lateral (*bottom*) radiographs immediately postoperative, showing a well-aligned ankle mortise with proper contouring of the talar allograft seated on the medial shoulder of the talus.

defect with subsequent cystic changes measuring 13 mm × 13 mm × 8 mm. Due to the CT findings and multiple failed conservative cares, it was decided to pursue excision of the lesion with bulk cadaveric talar allografting. This surgery took place 1 year and 10 months after the initial injury.

Access to the OCLT was gained through a medial malleolar osteotomy, as discussed previously (**Fig. 11**A). The pearl here is to complete the osteotomy with an osteotome to make a ridged contour to the osteotomy, allowing the medial malleolus to be reduced only in the correct manner at the end of the procedure (see **Fig. 11**A). The medial malleolus was reflected distally and the OCLT was promptly visualized (**Fig. 11**B). A marking pen then was used to draw out the clear margins of the OCLT in a cubed fashion (**Fig. 11**C). The OCLT then was removed and inspection taken to ensure no cystic lesion remains (**Fig. 11**D). On the back table, the allograft talus was prepared and secured down (**Fig. 11**E). The exact dimensions of the defect then were drawn out on the talar allograft. Once the proper sized allograft was obtained, it was placed into the talar defect created by removing the OCLT and secured in place with minifragment recessed or headless screws inserted medial to lateral (**Fig. 11**F). The medial malleolus then was reduced and fixated properly (**Fig. 11**G). Postoperative radiographs showed a well-aligned ankle mortise and proper contouring of the medial shoulder of the talus (**Fig. 12**).

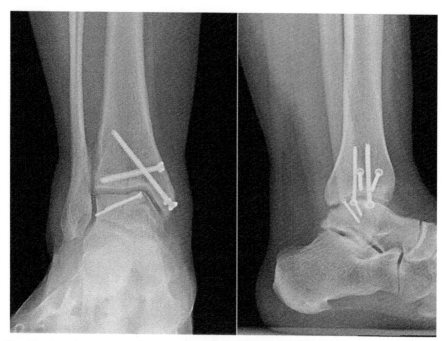

Fig. 13. .Anterior-posterior (*left*) and lateral (*right*) radiographs, indicating a fully incorporated talar allograft on the medial shoulder at 2-year follow-up.

The patient had an uneventfully recovery and began weight bearing at the 8-week mark in a fixed Anklizer boot (Bird and Cronin Inc, Eagan, MN). The patient progressed to full weight bearing and walking up to a mile per day with no pain at the 6-month mark, and, by a year out from surgery, the patient was able to return to her work without restrictions or bracing. The patient was seen at her 2-year follow-up with radiographs taken (**Fig. 13**). At her follow-up, she had been working at her job full time for a year without any setbacks and able to fully perform all activities she was able to prior to surgery without reservation or symptoms.

SUMMARY

Osteochondral lesions of the talus are a common pathology seen in a foot and ankle surgeon's practice and can prove a difficult problem to treat without the correct treatment algorithm. This article aims to provide an overview of OCLT, including imaging modalities for diagnosis and classification based on those findings. The treatments, both nonsurgical and surgical, are reviewed along with the treatment algorithm recommended by the authors. OCLTs can be treated in a variety of ways and patient factors along with the procedure that works best in the surgeon's hands should be taken into consideration as well as the size/stage of the OCLT. The cases reviewed provide evidence of the proposed treatments and techniques utilized that not only have proved successful to the authors but also demonstrate the potential complications that should be discussed with patients prior to surgery.

DISCLOSURE

The authors have nothing to disclose.

REFERENCES

1. Kraeutler MJ, Chahla J, Dean CS, et al. Current concepts review update: osteochondral lesions of the talus. Foot Ankle Int 2017;38(3):331–42.
2. Orr JD, Dawson LK, Garcia ESJ, et al. Incidence of osteochondral lesions of the talus in the United States military. Foot Ankle Int 2011;32(10):948–54.
3. Savage-Elliott I, Ross KA, Smyth NA, et al. Osteochondral lesions of the talus: a current concepts review and evidence-based treatment paradigm. Foot Ankle Spec 2014;7(5):414–22.
4. Schachter AK, Chen AL, Reddy PD, et al. Osteochondral lesions of the talus. J Am Acad Orthop Surg 2005;13(3):152–8.
5. Santrock R, Mathew B, Lee T, et al. Osteochondral lesions of the talus. Foot Ankle Clin N Am 2003;8:73–90.
6. Raikin SM, Elias I, Zoga AC, et al. Osteochondral lesions of the talus: localization and morphologic data from 424 patients using a novel anatomical grid scheme. Foot & ankle international 2007;28(2):154–61.
7. Elias I, Zoga AC, Morrison WB, et al. Osteochondral lesions of the talus: localization and morphologic data from 424 patients using a novel anatomical grid scheme. Foot Ankle Int 2007;28(2):154–61.
8. Takao M, Ochi M, Uchio Y, et al. Osteochondral lesions of the talar dome associated with truama. The J. Arthrscopic Related Surgery 2003;19(10):1061–7.
9. Verhagen RAW, Maas M, Dijkgraaf MGW, et al. Prospective study on diagnostic strategies in osteochondral lesions of the talus: is MRI superior to helical CT? J Bone Joint Surg Br 2005;87(1):41–6.
10. Looze CA, Capo J, Ryan MK, et al. Evaluation and management of osteochondral lesions of the talus. Cartilage 2017;8(1):19–30.
11. Joshy S, Abdulkadir U, Chaganti S, et al. Accuracy of MRI scan in the diagnosis of ligamentous and chondral pathology in the ankle. Foot Ankle Surg 2010;16(2):78–80.
12. Elias I, Jung JW, Raikin SM, et al. Osteochondral lesions of the talus: change in MRI findings over time in talar lesions without operative intervention and implications for staging systems. Foot Ankle Int 2006;27(3):157–66.
13. Van der Wall H, Lee A, Magee M, et al. Radionuclide bone scintigraphy in sports injuries. Semin Nucl Med 2010;40(No. 1):16–30. WB Saunders.
14. Meftah M, Katchis SD, Scharf SC, et al. SPECT/CT in the management of osteochondral lesions of the talus. Foot Ankle Int 2011;32(3):233–8.
15. Berndt A, Harty M. Transchondral fractures (osteochondritis dissecans) of the talus. J Bone Joint Surg Am 1959;41:988–1020.
16. Dipaola JD, Nelson DW, Colville MR. Characterizing osteochondral lesions by magnetic resonance imagin G. Arthroscopy 1991;7(1):101–4.
17. Hepple S, Winson IG, Glew D. Osteochondral lesions of the talus: a revised classification. Foot Ankle Int 1999;20(12):789–93.
18. Ferkel R, Sgaglione N, DelPizzo W. Arthroscopic treatment of osteochondral lesions of the talus: long-term results. Orthop Trans 1990;14:172–3.
19. Dahmen J, Lambers KT, Reilingh ML, et al. No superior treatment for primary osteochondral defects of the talus. Knee Surg Sports Traumatol Arthrosc 2018;26(7):2142–57.
20. Zengerink M, Struijs PA, Tol JL, et al. Treatment of osteochondral lesions of the talus: a systematic review. Knee Surg Sports Traumatol Arthrosc 2010;18(2):238–46.

21. Tol JL, Struijs PAA, Bossuyt PMM, et al. Treatment strategies in osteochondral defects of the talar dome: a systematic review. Foot Ankle Int 2000;21(2):119–26.
22. Chuckpaiwong B, Berkson EM, Theodore GH. Microfracture for osteochondral lesions of the ankle: outcome analysis and outcome predictors of 105 cases. Arthroscopy 2008;24(1):106–12.
23. van Bergen CJ, de Leeuw PA, van Dijk CN. Potential pitfall in the microfracturing technique during the arthroscopic treatment of an osteochondral lesion. Knee Surg Sports Traumatol Arthrosc 2009;17(2):184–7.
24. Murawski CD, Kennedy JG. Operative treatment of osteochondral lesions of the talus. J Bone Joint Surg Am 2013;95(11):1045–54.
25. Donnenwerth MP, Roukis TS. Outcome of arthroscopic debridement and microfracture as the primary treatment for osteochondral lesions of the talar dome. Arthroscopy 2012;28(12):1902–7.
26. Cuttica DJ, Smith WB, Hyer CF, et al. Osteochondral lesions of the talus: predictors of clinical outcome. Foot Ankle Int 2011;32(11):1045–51.
27. Lui TH. Arthroscopic bone grafting of talar bone cyst using posterior ankle arthroscopy. J Foot Ankle Surg 2013;52(4):529–32.
28. McWilliams GD, Yao L, Simonet LB, et al. Subchondroplasty of the ankle and hindfoot for treatment of osteochondral lesions and stress fractures: initial imaging experience. Foot Ankle Spec 2019. https://doi.org/10.1177/1938640019863252.
29. Hangody L, Ráthonyi GK, Duska Z, et al. Autologous osteochondral mosaicplasty: surgical technique. J Bone Joint Surg Am 2004;86(suppl_1):65–72.
30. Adams SB, Dekker TJ, Schiff AP, et al. Prospective evaluation of structural allograft transplantation for osteochondral lesions of the talar shoulder. Foot Ankle Int 2018;39(1):28–34.
31. Orr JD, Dunn JC, Heida KA Jr, et al. Results and functional outcomes of structural fresh osteochondral allograft transfer for treatment of osteochondral lesions of the talus in a highly active population. Foot Ankle Spec 2017;10(2):125–32.
32. VanTienderen RJ, Dunn JC, Kusnezov N, et al. Osteochondral allograft transfer for treatment of osteochondral lesions of the talus: a systematic review. Arthroscopy 2017;33(1):217–22.
33. Easley ME, Latt DL, Santangelo JR, et al. Osteochondral lesions of the talus. J Am Acad Orthop Surg 2010;18(10):616–30.
34. Roukis TS, Kang RB. Vascularized pedicled fibula onlay bone graft augmentation for complicated tibiotalocalcaneal arthrodesis with retrograde intramedullary nail fixation: a case series. J Foot Ankle Surg 2016;55(4):857–67.
35. Rogero R, Tsai J, Shakked R, et al. Mid-term results of radiographic and functional outcomes after tibiotalocalcaneal arthrodesis with bulk femoral head allograft. Foot & Ankle Orthopaedics 2018;3(3). 2473011418S00408.

Revision Surgery for the Achilles Tendon

Amber M. Shane, DPM[a],*, Christopher L. Reeves, DPM[a], Garrett B. Nguyen, DPM[b], Joshua A. Sebag, DPM[b]

KEYWORDS

- Revisional Achilles tendon • Reconstruction • Augmentation
- Gastrocnemius lengthening • Turndown flap • Tendon transfer • Autografts
- Allografts

KEY POINTS

- Surgical management for the revisional Achilles tendon is complex and often involves a multifactorial approach with advanced repair options.
- A gastrocnemius lengthening or fascial turndown may be performed to assist in end-to-end repair where difficulty is encountered with reapproximation of tissue ends or not feasible because of loss of length.
- When indicated, flexor hallucis longus transfer should be used as the tendon transfer of choice to supplement the pull of the native Achilles tendon.
- Avoid more than 15° of dorsiflexion when tensioning repair; frequently 5° of correction are lost because of contracture and adhesions.
- Meticulous layered closure is vital to prevent postoperative wound complications.

INTRODUCTION

Rupture of the Achilles tendon is a common tendon disorder encountered by foot and ankle surgeons, with a reported annual incidence of 18 ruptures per 100,000 people.[1] First reported by Ambroise Paré in 1575, treatment remained primarily nonsurgical until the twentieth century. It was not until Abrahamson in 1923, and later Queru and Staianovich in 1929, that surgical treatment of the ruptured Achilles tendon began to gain momentum.[2]

Treatment of Achilles tendon ruptures may be surgical or nonsurgical depending on the acuity and severity of the injury. However, with chronic or revisional injuries, the best method often requires an open repair with reconstructive soft tissue procedures.

[a] Advent Health East Orlando Podiatric Surgery Residency, Orlando Foot and Ankle Clinic-Upperline Health, 250 North Alafaya Trail Suite 115, Orlando, FL 32828, USA; [b] Department of Podiatric Surgery, Advent Health East Orlando Podiatric Surgery Residency, 250 North Alafaya Trail Suite 1115, Orlando, FL 32828, USA
* Corresponding author.
E-mail address: Ashane@orlandofoot.com

Clin Podiatr Med Surg 37 (2020) 553–568
https://doi.org/10.1016/j.cpm.2020.03.005
0891-8422/20/© 2020 Elsevier Inc. All rights reserved.

Revision surgery for the Achilles tendon can pose a challenge to many surgeons because of the complexity involving large tendinous deficits with nonviable and friable tissue. This challenge can be further complicated by increased time to treatment or delay of treatment. With revisional Achilles tendon disorders, several anatomic changes occur, such as retraction of tendon ends and fatty infiltration, which can necessitate further debridement of the tendon ends and lead to a larger deficit.[1] Complication rates of Achilles tendon repair tend to be low, although traditional risk factors, such as corticosteroid use, smoking, delay in treatment, and diabetes, can all influence complication rates.[3] Further, even in cases where the revisional Achilles tendon repair healed well, there is often a concern for the surrounding soft tissue envelope to heal without complication. This concern may add some inherent risk when surgeons are addressing a hostile skin region where a thick scar may already be present.

ANATOMY

The Achilles tendon is the largest and strongest tendon in the body, and acts as the primary plantarflexor of the ankle. It is a conjoined tendon consisting of the gastrocnemius and soleus muscles, with a small contribution of the plantaris muscle, and is located in the superficial posterior compartment of the calf. Approximately 15 cm long, the tendon begins at the musculotendinous junction of the gastrocnemius and soleus and extends to its insertion onto the middle of the posterior surface of the calcaneus. This roughened ridge is best suited for osteotendinous attachment.

Rather than a true synovial sheath, the tendon is enclosed within a paratenon that acts as a thin gliding membrane. The blood supply to the Achilles tendon is provided through its musculotendinous junction via the paratenon through transversely oriented vincula that act as passageways to aid on vascular delivery.[4] It is also supplied directly from its bone insertion to the calcaneus. The vascular supply is divided into 3 regions, with the midsection being supplied by the peroneal artery, whereas the proximal and distal portions are supplied by the posterior tibial artery.[5] The area of lowest vascularity within the tendon is located 2 cm to 6 cm above its insertion.[6] This pattern of blood supply, along with the anatomic spiraling of the tendon, may contribute to the pathogenesis of Achilles tendon injury, through overuse and rupture. This area has been suggested as a relative watershed zone because of the imbalance of perfusion to collagen. Blood supply to the tendon may also decrease with age, and this poor vascularity may lead to weakening of the tendon, predispose to injury, and inhibit tissue repair after trauma.

INCIDENCE

Reruptures and complications following Achilles tendon repairs are uncommon, with rates ranging from 1.7% to 5.6% within the literature.[7] A 2018 retrospective review by Jildeh and colleagues[3] studied 423 patients undergoing surgical treatment, and revealed a 1% rerupture rate and a 2.8% overall infection rate, with correlations associated with longer operative times. It is generally thought that the risk of rerupture is highest within the first 2 months following the end of nonoperative treatment, although there is little high-level evidence to support this notion.[8] Other studies have shown that risk of rerupture is highest following termination of cast or orthosis treatment in nonoperative protocols.[8] Other studies failed to correlate type of immobilization, time to treatment, cause of rupture, gender, sporting and nonsporting individuals, or immunosuppressive treatment with increased risk of rerupture.[9,10]

CAUSE

Reasons for revision surgery for the Achilles tendon can be broadly divided into wound breakdown caused by infection, delayed/nonhealing of the soft tissue and skin, or rerupture/gapping of the tendon. Although these complications may have distinct causes, surgical management and treatment of these complications are not mutually exclusive. Often, surgeons have to find a solution for all 3 reasons because they can progress in a stepwise fashion from wound breakdown with subsequent infection and skin necrosis to gapping of the Achilles tendon secondary to surgical debridement of nonviable tissue.

Many histopathologic changes occur with regard to the chronic/revisional Achilles tendon. Native, uninjured Achilles tendon typically consist of more than 90% parallel bundles of type I collagen.[6] However, in a tendon that has been ruptured or tendinopathic, the tenocytes produce higher proportions of type 3 collagen, leading to a decrease in tensile force.[11,12] With strain levels greater than 8%, disruptions in the intermolecular crosslinks become problematic, resulting in tensile failure and macroscopic rupture and breakdown.[6,13] A study by Tallon and colleagues[14] echoed these findings when they evaluated histologic differences between ruptured and unruptured Achilles tendon. They found alterations in the ruptured Achilles tendon that showed a decrease in collagen organization, increase in collagen degeneration, and an imbalance of increased extracellular matrix with decreased collagen fiber. In turn, the combination of these characteristics resulted in the tendon being less resistant to tensile forces, predisposing to reruptures and injury. Other reported causes include fluoroquinolones, angiotensin II receptor antagonists, corticosteroid-induced collagen necrosis, gout, arteriosclerosis, hyperthyroidism, tobacco use, diabetes, and renal insufficiency.[15–19]

DIAGNOSIS AND PREOPERATIVE PLANNING

A thorough history and physical is paramount when evaluating for Achilles tendon disorders or ruptures. On physical examination, a palpable gap or dell may be felt along the course of the Achilles tendon, often in conjunction with some calf muscle wasting with pain. Manual muscle testing may reveal decreased plantarflexory power in the affected limb with an increase in dorsiflexory moment.

Historically, several diagnostic tests have been proposed in the literature to assess for any disruption in the Achilles tendon. These tests include the notable Thompson calf-squeeze test, knee-flexion test, and the less used needle and sphygmomanometer test.[20–23] Other diagnostic methods, such as MRI or ultrasonography, can help determine the extent of the defect or gap size, which is necessary for preoperative planning.[24] In conjunction, viability of other tendons, such as the flexor hallucis longus (FHL), can be ascertained if planning for tendon transfers.

TREATMENT

Treatment with revision surgery of the Achilles tendon requires a multifactorial approach. Surgeons should follow a step-by-step algorithm and guide for the management of wound breakdown, infection, and rerupture after Achilles tendon surgery. Infection must be cleared and debridement of all nonviable tissue performed before assessment of the tendon quality can be measured. If primary repair without tendon defect is possible, closure of the wound with protection of the posterior soft tissue is performed. If repaired, but tendon strength is weakened, tendon transfers may be performed. When reapproximation is not feasible, procedures, including gastrocnemius aponeurosis lengthening or turndown procedures, can be performed. In addition, for large tendon deficits, autografts or allografts may be used in conjunction with the previously mentioned methods to bridge and repair complicated revisional cases.

Classically, Myerson[25] outlined an algorithm for the repair of the neglected Achilles tendon rupture. Achilles tendon ruptures with defects spanning 1 to 2 cm can be repaired with a simple end-to-end anastomosis. For defects spanning 2 to 5 cm, it is recommended that a V-Y myotendinous lengthening be performed in conjunction with an end-to-end anastomosis. Consideration of a FHL transfer may be warranted for defects with considerable nonviable tissue. For defects larger than 5 cm, Myerson[25] advocates the use of turndown flaps in conjunction with the previously mentioned surgical techniques for the repair of neglected Achilles tendon ruptures. In addition, for defects larger than 5 cm, it is recommended that an FHL tendon transfer be used as the first option.

Given the infrequency of these complications, definitive literature evidence guiding treatment is highly debated. Surgical treatment recommendations guided by defect size can be seen in **Table 1** after infection is eliminated, if present, and proper debridement of all nonviable soft tissue obtained. Treatment options tend to mirror protocols for chronic ruptures of the Achilles because there is a general lack of consensus in evaluations of the treatment of revisional Achilles tendon. As such, many of the principles guiding treatment of chronic ruptures can be applied to the revision surgery of the Achilles tendon with favorable outcomes. These principles include end-to-end repairs, gastrocnemius-soleus lengthenings, fascial turndowns, tendon transfers, autografts, and allografts. This article presents evidence-based surgical techniques and data for the revisional Achilles tendon.

End-to-End Anastomosis

Ultimately, the simplest and most efficient way to reapproximate the torn Achilles is by end-to-end anastomosis (**Figs. 1** and **2**). In the case of revisional or neglected Achilles ruptures, complete debridement of degenerative tissues with poor healing potential is often required. Interestingly, a direct repair technique using part of the interposed scar tissue for revisional ruptures has been described with good functional and clinical outcomes.[26] By resecting only the middle portion of the scar tissue and interposing the remaining scar tissue between the tendon stumps, direct repair of revisional Achilles tendon ruptures is possible without the use of autografts or allografts.

Table 1 Surgical treatment of the revisional Achilles tendon	
Defect Size	**Recommended Treatment/ Procedure**
<2 cm with viable tendon integrity	End-to-end repair ±V-Y lengthening
<2 cm with nonviable tendon integrity	End-to-end repair with FHL transfer ±V-Y lengthening
2–5 cm	V-Y lengthening ±FHL transfer ±Turndown advancement
>5 cm	Turndown advancement ±FHL transfer ±Autograft/allograft

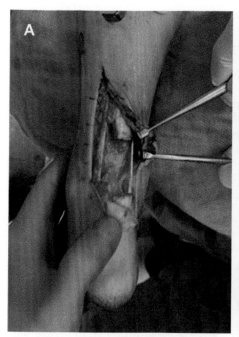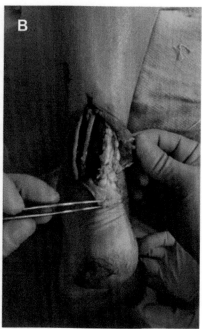

Fig. 1. (*A*) Complete debridement of degenerated tendon following complex laceration repair. (*B*) End-to-end repair using Krackow stitch with plantaris tendon augmentation.

Although the Krackow stitch is the most common direct repair technique, variations have been widely described. A biomechanical study conducted by Mckeon and colleagues[27] found that an additional second interlocking suture placed at 90° to the first suture was nearly twice as strong as a single interlocking suture when comparing peak load to failure: 290 N versus 534 N. In addition, Hong and colleagues[28] found that Krackow stitch intervals of 2.5 and 5.0 mm showed a significantly smaller tendon elongation (31% and 32%) compared with an interval of 10.0 mm (41%). Regarding new suture constructs for end-to-end repairs, White and colleagues[29] found no significant difference in construct elongation when comparing the traditional Krackow stitch with premanufactured locking loop stitch for soft tissue fixation. Overall, consideration of tendon quality, apposition feasibility, and reapproximation technique must all be scrutinized for proper revisional repair.

Gastrocnemius-Soleus Lengthening

Many procedures have been described to lengthen the gastrocnemius-soleus complex. With revision surgery for Achilles tendon ruptures, large deficits often require a combination of procedures, including gastrocnemius lengthenings, to reapproximate gapped tendon stumps. Herzenberg and colleagues[30] in 2007 evaluated the effects of an isolated Baumann procedure on 15 normal cadavers. Their study showed that the Baumann isolates the lengthening site to the gastrocnemius muscle belly without lengthening the soleus muscle. Although not routinely performed, the procedure preserves muscle strength while providing intramuscular lengthening.

More commonly performed for the reduction of gastrocnemius equinus deformities, a Strayer may also be used in order to achieve apposition of tendon stumps. Because of its inherent vascularity directly adjacent to the well-perfused gastrocnemius muscle

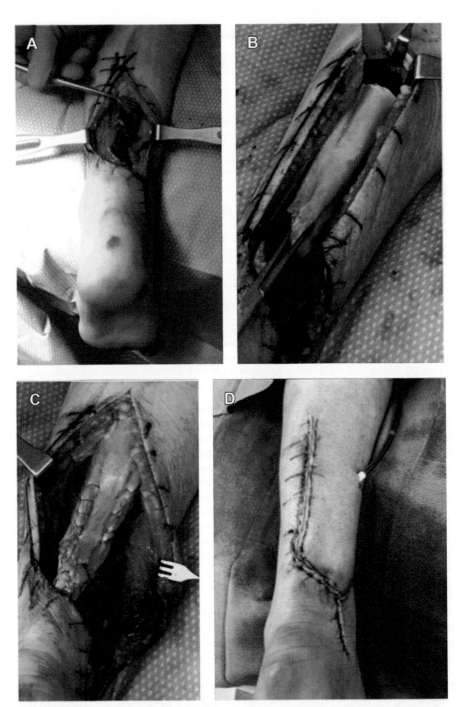

Fig. 2. Complex posterior leg and tendon laceration treated with debridement (*A*), gastrocnemius aponeurosis lengthening (*B*), and end-to-end repair (*C*). Note the addition of a drain to help mitigate both the risk of hematoma formation and undesirable pressures at the site of closure (*D*).

bellies, complications regarding this lengthening are acceptably low. Other lengthening procedures include the Baker or Vulpius, which allow a greater release and lengthening of the combined gastrocnemius-soleus complex and therefore a more fluid and complete lengthening.

For deficits up to 5 cm, Abraham and Pankovich[31] in 1975 originally described a V-Y advancement for end-to-end repairs of Achilles ruptures. By approximating the arms of the V incision to correspond with 1.5 times the length of the defect, large closures were possible.[31] Variations of the Bosworth V-Y technique for chronic ruptures have also been used with success in revisional surgery of the Achilles. Nilsson-Helander and colleagues[32] in 2008 described a free gastrocnemius aponeurosis flap for reruptures and chronic ruptures in 28 patients, 15 of which were reruptures. This method rendered a good outcome by both subjective and objective measures in both patient cohorts. Nonetheless, several studies have cited disadvantages of isolated V-Y advancements.[33–35] Us and colleagues[33] noted a 22% decrease in peak torque when using isolated V-Y lengthening. Similarly, Kissel and colleagues[34] revealed a 30% decrease in functional power with the same procedure. Elais and colleagues[35] in 2007 reiterated these concerns and recommended augmenting such a procedure with an FHL transfer to improve plantarflexory power. This recommendation supports the notion of combination procedures where necessary to optimize patient outcomes.

Fascial Turndown

In the case of large tendon deficits (>5 cm) with profound muscle wasting and stump retraction, fascial turndown procedures are often indicated to supplement gastrocnemius lengthenings and tendon transfers. Bosworth[36] in 1956 noted that, by bridging gap deficits with healthy viable tendon, reformation of normal tendon from the interposed remnants was possible. Originally described using a central portion of the tendoachilles complex, the resected tendon was flapped downward and imbricated transversely across the distal stump and back into the proximally stump to be sutured onto itself.[36] Lee and colleagues[37] in 2005 described a modified Bosworth technique that sutured the end into the proximal stump in patients with insufficient length. All patients returned to normal ambulation without major complications involving rerupture, deep infection, skin necrosis, or persistent equinus.

However, because of the increase in soft tissue volume at the repair site, complications involving wound dehiscence have been reported.[38] Khiami and colleagues[38] in 2013 proposed a modified technique of implementing a free sural triceps aponeurosis harvested proximally and transposed between the diseased tendon after performing a Z-plasty. Their technique not only reduced soft tissue thickness thereby negating the associated complication risks but also allowed for length adjustments to be made when repairing. Mean American Orthopaedic Foot and Ankle Society (AOFAS) score was 96, with 12 of 16 patients returning to sport. MRI evaluation taken at 1 year postoperatively revealed homogeneous tendon and graft integration along with an increase in tendon size. These findings presented acceptable clinical results with this technique.

Similarly, Guclu and colleagues[39] in 2017 examined a modified V-Y approach using a fascial turndown in 17 patients at a mean of 7 months from the time of injury. They found a mean AOFAS score of 95 postoperatively over a mean follow-up of 16 years with a rerupture rate of 0%.[39]

Other variations of the turndown procedure have been detailed in the literature, including the Lindholm technique, with equivocal results[40,41] (**Fig. 3**). Repairs implementing fascial turndown techniques allow earlier mobility, weight bearing, and often

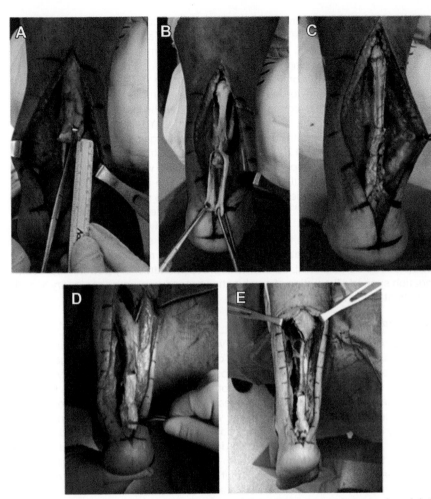

Fig. 3. (*A*) Measurement of the Achilles tendon deficit is performed after complete debridement of all nonviable tendon. (*B*) Lindholm turndown flap is made using a medial and lateral technique. (*C*) Complete repair of the distal turndown flap. (*D*) A modified Lindholm turndown flap can be made via a single-flap technique. At least 1 cm of native tendon is left attached at the soft tissue hinge to reduce tearing. (*E*) V-Y, modified Vulpius, can be seen sutured, providing additional tendon length.

more aggressive rehabilitation protocols, thereby reducing complications in the surgical treatment of revisional Achilles tendons.[42]

Tendon Transfer

Tendon transfers have been well described in the literature to augment the repair of acute, chronic, and revisional Achilles tendon ruptures. The most commonly used tendons include the plantaris, peroneus brevis (PB), peroneus longus, flexor digitorum longus (FDL), and FHL.

Plantaris

Although the plantaris tendon is considered the easiest to harvest, pathophysiologic changes in a chronic or revisional Achilles tendon can often provide a challenge for surgeons. This tendon is usually heavily incorporated within the diseased Achilles tendon and may be difficult to identify and dissect away. However, if identified, it does possess the advantage of being harmoniously functional with the Achilles tendon. It also provides substantial autograft potential to reconstructive surgeons.

Akgun and colleagues[43] in 2006 documented a case study that combined the plantaris tendon to augment the treatment of the Achilles tendon rupture. Sedek and colleagues[44] in 2015 described a surgical technique using the plantaris tendon to create a triple loop for the repair of Achilles tendon ruptures larger than 5 cm. In this case series, 18 patients with Myerson type III rupture were enrolled. The technique involved harvesting the plantaris proximally and fashioning a triple loop connecting the proximal and distal ends of the Achilles tendon and anchoring the distal end into a calcaneal drill hole. The plantaris tendon was then overlapped by the lateral half of a turndown flap. Results reached statistical significance when evaluating the Achilles tendon for healing and gap disappearance. The mean preoperative AOFAS was 62.2 points, whereas, at the patients' last follow-up, the mean postoperative score was 94.9 points.[44] In similar fashion, Jain and colleagues[45] in 2014 repaired defects larger than 2 cm using the free plantaris tendon graft in a circular configuration, encompassing the turndown flap, with comparable results.

Peroneus brevis

Peroneus brevis transfers have been described for both acute and chronic ruptures.[46] In a study by Nagakiran and colleagues,[47] the functional outcomes of FHL versus PB transfers for chronic ruptures were compared, and both cohorts were shown to have nearly identical AOFAS scores and Achilles Tendon Total Rupture (ATTR) scores. Concerns for functional deficit of eversion with transfer of the peroneus brevis are exaggerated, because the peroneus longus has double the eversion strength of its brevis counterpart.[48] Gallant and colleagues[49] in 1995 showed no functional compromise of the ankle joint or eversion with PB transfer. Pintore and colleagues[50] in 2001 performed a cohort study comparing PB transfer in chronic ruptures with acute ruptures with end-end anastomosis. Patients with this treatment were satisfied with the procedure but had higher complication rates and greater loss of strength than those with acute ruptures. The technique for this procedure typically entails freeing the insertion from the base of the fifth metatarsal, tagging with suture, passing through the posterior intermuscular septum, and anchoring through a medial-lateral transosseous hole or weaving through the Achilles tendon.[46]

Peroneus longus

In the setting of infection following Achilles tendon ruptures with concomitant FHL transfer, salvage procedures using the peroneus longus can be performed. Chan and colleagues[51] in 2013 described a case report of a peroneus longus transfer into the calcaneus with an interference screw to reconstruct a reruptured Achilles tendon. They found satisfactory results over an 18-month follow-up in terms of activity, resting tendon tension, and eversion strength. Similarly, Wang and colleagues[52] in 2009 harvested the peroneus longus through several stab incisions and fixated the tendon into the plantar calcaneus with a cortical button. At a 2.5-year follow-up, MRI revealed maintenance of the long peroneal within the calcaneal osseous tunnel and anatomic alignment of the Achilles tendon. No decrease in plantarflexion or hindfoot eversion was evident after active rehabilitation.

Flexor digitorum longus

FDL transfer represents another viable option for repair of the revisional Achilles tendon. This technique was first described by Mann and colleagues in 1991 and has since been shown in several studies to have adequate results with transfer.[53] Drawbacks include dissection in close proximity to the neurovascular bundle, as well as weaker plantarflexion strength and an increased distance from the Achilles than the FHL.[54] A similar tenotomy, tagging, and transosseous calcaneal placement with tendon weaving is used for this procedure.[54] If performing the FHL tendon transfer, surgeons must distinguish the FDL from the FHL because they may be easily confused. In almost all cases the FDL tendon is smaller than a native FHL.

Flexor hallucis longus

At present, the FHL tendon is considered the gold standard for transfer in cases of chronic and revisional surgery of Achilles tendon ruptures.[46] It is in phase with the Achilles tendon, serves as the second strongest plantar flexor in the lower extremity, and helps to perfuse the avascular zone of the Achilles with its distal muscle belly.[46] There are numerous ways to harvest the FHL for use. The most typical approach entails a single incision harvested through the posterior rearfoot[46] (**Fig. 4**). A double-incision technique has also been described, with the second midfoot incision just proximal to the knot of Henry. An average of an additional 3 cm can be obtained for longer tendon transfers and augmentation with this technique.[55] Avoiding violation of the knot of Henry maintains near-normal function of the FHL via a coordinated effort based on the pull of the adjacent FDL and joint tendinous attachments at the knot of Henry.

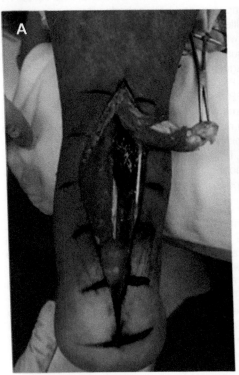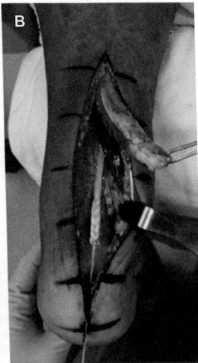

Fig. 4. (A) Achilles tendon following debridement is reflected proximally with the FHL visible underneath. (B) The FHL tendon has been harvested, whipstitched, and prepared for tenodesis to the calcaneus, which has been prepared with a power rasp for reapproximation of both tendons.

Goss and colleagues[56] in 2019 described a minimally invasive retrograde method in which they used a transverse plantar incision at the hallux interphalangeal joint and a tendon stripper to advance the tendon proximally for transfer. Graft length with this method averaged 13.3 cm, providing a longer graft than other approaches.[56] Vega and colleagues in 2018 described an endoscopic transfer for chronic ruptures, in which the technique was performed on 22 patients with excellent results.[57] However, the investigators noted that the procedure is technically challenging and is not recommended for surgeons that lack endoscopic experience.[57]

A plausible concern with the FHL transfer is loss of push-off strength and gait disturbance following harvest of the tendon. Coull and colleagues[58] in 2003 reviewed morbidity following FHL transfer and found insignificant changes in pedobarographic pressure, average AOFAS hallux score of 97, and negligible functional deficit of the hallux. Elias and colleagues[59] in 2009 examined corresponding results and noted that 92.5% of their patients at a 27-month follow-up were able to perform 20 single-heel raises on the surgical side with no clinical difference in strength compared with the nonoperative limb. Universally, there were no patients who reported gait disturbances or any decrease in hallux strength.

It is important to evaluate the bone-to-tendon interface because fixation must be stronger than the physiologic load applied, otherwise failure is inevitable. The original surgical technique involved passing the tendon through a transosseous drill hole in the posterior calcaneus and weaving the tendon through the Achilles.[46] However, this technique requires significant tendon length and therefore more distal tendon harvests. Other fixation techniques include use of an interference screw, cortical button, or a combination of all of them to obtain multiple fixation points.[60] Cortical buttons were found to be the strongest with respect to load to failure in multiple studies.[61–63] Even more surprising, constructs composed of an interference screw along with a cortical button produced the least displacement at the bone-to-tendon interface compared with an interference screw or cortical button alone.[64] For this reason, fixation of an FHL transfer should ideally include both a plantar cortical button and inference screw.

Beyond clinical outcomes, a study by Hahn and colleagues[65] examined tendon incorporation of the FHL on MRI at 3.8 years' follow-up after transfer. Twelve of 13 tendons showed a significant degree of incorporation, and FHL muscle belly showed an average increase in size of 17%. The occurrence of both tendon incorporation and muscle belly hypertrophy revealed a functional adaptive ability of the FHL tendon with regard to transfer to the Achilles.[65]

Autografts

Other autografts and transfers have gained popularity in recent years as augmentation options for chronic or revisional Achilles tendon ruptures have become more available. Maffulli and colleagues[66] in 2014 described a minimally invasive free semitendinosus graft for reconstruction of chronic deficits. This technique was performed on 28 patients with good to excellent results in 93% and 57% returning to preinjury level of sport.[66] Patil and colleagues[67] in 2014 treated 35 chronic ruptures with an open technique that harvested the semitendinosus tendon with satisfactory functional outcome and no reruptures.

Numerous other reconstructive options have also been well described, including local and regional flaps to transpositional free flaps. Often, microvascular anastomosis must be performed for flap survival, and these are technically more demanding. In these cases, soft tissue coverage and closure are difficult to obtain. Kelahmetoglu and colleagues[68] in 2017 repaired a complex revisional Achilles tendon rupture with a free composite anterolateral thigh flap with vascularized fascia lata. Preoperative and postoperative AOFAS scores were 11 and 98, respectively. Visual analog scales of pain decreased from 8 to 1. No complications were reported and the patient was able to return to daily ambulating activity without support within 5 months.

Donor site morbidity and functionality should always be assessed. As with any autograft harvesting, a second incision is required. Given the patient's age, comorbidities, and functional status, autografts and transfers may be a viable option when indicated.

Allografts

For large defects (>5 cm) with friable or nonviable tissues at the distal Achilles stump, or when adjacent host tissues are not suited for tissue transfer, it is acceptable that Achilles tendon allografts with or without bone blocks be used. With severe degeneration at the insertion of the bone-to-tendon interface, use of bone blocks is essential. Bone blocks should be shaped and measured according to the patient's calcaneus and fixated.

Cienfuegos and colleagues[69] reported a reconstruction of a 12-cm deficit using an Achilles tendon allograft. Outcomes revealed no limitations to performing bilateral heel raise at 3 months, with full return to activity at 1 year. Lepow and Green[70] also reported a reconstruction of a 10-cm deficit using an Achilles tendon allograft with similar outcomes: bilateral heel rise at 10 weeks with return to prefunctional capacity at 1-year follow-up.

Deese and colleagues[71] retrospectively reviewed 8 patients with deficits ranging from 5.5 cm to 10 cm. All repairs were made with an Achilles tendon allograft with a calcaneal bone block. At final follow-up visit, no pain or reruptures were reported, with good functional outcomes. Minor complications included delayed healing to the incision and heterotopic bone formation in the retrocalcaneal bursa. Comparably, Ofili and colleagues[72] performed a retrospective review of 14 cases, 2 of which used an Achilles tendon allograft with calcaneal bone block. Deficits ranged from 4 to 15 cm with single heel rise at 12 and 37 weeks respectively. Complications included delayed union of the calcaneal bone block. No reruptures were reported. All maintained good functional and clinical outcomes at final visit.

SUMMARY

There are numerous ways to approach revisional Achilles tendon rupture surgery, despite a paucity of information regarding the subject in the literature. Surgical approaches are challenging and complex because tissues are degenerated, often leaving significant deficits once debrided. Tendon retraction, adhesions, and muscular wasting are also evident, making simple primary repair techniques more difficult. The goal of treatment is to restore anatomic and physiologic tension, provide adequate strength for proper ambulation, optimize functional return to activity, and decrease the recurrence and complications associated with revisional surgery. A variety of techniques are available within the surgeon's toolbox, with a general consensus of operative management in these cases. Functional outcomes are statistically superior when comparing operative versus nonoperative techniques in the revisional setting. Surgical techniques are primarily dictated by deficit size, tendon integrity, and functional demands. Techniques include end-to-end repair, gastrocnemius-soleus lengthenings, fascial turndowns, tendon transfers, as well as supplemental grafting.

A gastrocnemius lengthening or fascial turndown may be performed to assist in end-to-end repair where difficulty is encountered with reapproximation of tissue ends. When indicated, FHL transfer should be used to supplement the pull of the native Achilles tendon. Fixation for the tendon transfer should include both a plantar cortical button and inference screw. For defects larger than 5 cm with friable, nonviable soft tissue, or absence of soft tissue coverage, the use of autografts/allografts can provide an indispensable option. As with all surgical incisions, meticulous dissection, hemostasis, and closure are vital to avoiding devastating complications. If possible, anterior-based splints can be applied to reduce posterior wound and pressure complications. In order to achieve optimal surgical outcomes, proper postoperative care and appropriately timed physical therapy are essential. Ultimately, surgical management for revisional Achilles tendon is complex and often involves a multifactorial approach with advanced repair options. Surgeons should always use their own discretion and expertise when treating such cases.

DISCLOSURE

The authors have nothing to disclose.

REFERENCES

1. Krahe M, Berlet GC. Achilles tendon ruptures, re rupture with revision surgery, tendinosis and insertional disease. Foot Ankle Clin 2009;14(2):247–75.
2. Cetti R, Christensen SE. Surgical treatment under local anesthesia of Achilles tendon rupture. Clin Orthop 1983;173:204–8.
3. Jildeh TR, Okoroha KR, Marshall NE, et al. Infection and rerupture after surgical repair of achilles tendons. Orthop J Sports Med 2018;6(5). 2325967118774302.
4. Maffulli N, Sharma P, Luscombe KL. Achilles tendinopathy: aetiology and management. J R Soc Med 2004;97(10):472–6.
5. Doral M, Alam M, Bozkurt M, et al. Functional anatomy of the Achilles tendon. Knee Surg Sports Traumatol Arthrosc 2010;18. https://doi.org/10.1007/s00167-010-1083-7.
6. O'Brien M. The anatomy of the Achilles tendon. Foot Ankle Clin N Am 2005;10:225–38.
7. Hanada M, Takahashi M, Matsuyama Y. Open re-rupture of the Achilles tendon after surgical treatment. Clin Pract 2011;1(4):e134.
8. Reito A, Logren H-L, Ahonen K, et al. Risk factors for failed nonoperative treatment and rerupture in acute achilles tendon rupture. Foot Ankle Int 2018;39(6):694–703.
9. Ingvar J, Tagil M, Eneroth M. Nonoperative treatment of Achilles tendon rupture: 196 consecutive patients with a 7% re-rupture rate. Acta Orthop 2005;76(4):597–601.
10. Wallace RG, Heyes GJ, Michael AL. The non-operative functional management of patients with a rupture of the tendo Achillis leads to low rates of re-rupture. J Bone Joint Surg Br 2011;93(10):1362–6.
11. Maffulli N, Ewen SW, Waterston SW, et al. Tenocytes from ruptured and tendinopathic Achilles tendons produce greater quantities of type III collagen than tenocytes from normal Achilles tendons. An in vitro model of human tendon healing. Am J Sports Med 2000;28:499–505.
12. Strocchi R, De Pasquale V, Guizzardi S, et al. Human Achilles tendon: morphological and morphometric variations as a function of age. Foot Ankle 1991;12:100–4.
13. Maganaris CN, Narici MN, Maffulli N. Biomechanics of the achilles tendon. Disabil Rehabil 2008;30:1542–7.

14. Tallon C, Maffulli N, Ewen SW. Ruptured Achilles tendons are significantly more degenerated than tendinopathic tendons. Med Sci Sports Exerc 2001;33: 1983–90.

15. Nyyssönen T, Lantto I, Lüthje P, et al. Drug treatments associated with achilles tendon rupture. A case-control study involving 1118 achilles tendon ruptures. Scand J Med Sci Sports 2018;28(12):2625–9.

16. Hersh BL, Heath NS. Achilles tendon rupture as a result of oral steroid therapy. J Am Podiatric Med Assoc 2002;92(6):355–8.

17. Mahoney PG, James PD, Howell CJ, et al. Spontaneous rupture of the achilles tendon in a patient with gout. Ann Rheum Dis 1981;40(4):416–8.

18. Petersen W, Pufe T, Zantop T, et al. Expression of VEGFR1 and VEGFR-2 in degenerative Achilles tendons. Clin Orthop Relat Res 2004;420:286–91.

19. Thevendran G, Sarraf KM, Patel NK, et al. The ruptured achilles tendon: a current overview from biology of rupture to treatment. Musculoskelet Surg 2013; 97(1):9–20.

20. Thompson TC. A test for rupture of the tendo Achillis. Acta Orthop Scand 1962; 32:461–5.

21. Matles AL. Rupture of the tendo Achilles: another diagnostic sign. Bull Hosp Joint Dis 1975;36:48–51.

22. O'Brien T. The needle test for complete rupture of the Achilles tendon. J Bone Joint Surg 1984;66A:1099–101.

23. Copeland SA. Rupture of the Achilles tendon: a new clinical test. Ann R Coll Surg Engl 1990;72:270–1.

24. Padanilam TG. Chronic Achilles tendon ruptures. Foot Ankle Clin 2009;14(4): 711–28.

25. Myerson MS. Achilles tendon rupture. Instr Course Lect 1999;48:226–7.

26. Yasuda T, Shima H, Mori K, et al. Direct repair of chronic achilles tendon ruptures using scar tissue located between the tendon stumps. J Bone Joint Surg 2016; 98(14):1168–75.

27. Mckeon BP, Heming JF, Fulkerson J, et al. The Krackow Stitch: a biomechanical evaluation of changing the number of loops versus the number of sutures. Arthroscopy 2006;22(1):33–7.

28. Hong C-K, Lin C-L, Kuan F-C, et al. Longer Stitch Interval in the Krackow Stitch for tendon graft fixation leads to poorer biomechanical property. J Orthopaedic Surg 2018;26(3). 2309499018799951.

29. White KL, Camire LM, Parks BG, et al. Krackow locking stitch versus locking pre-manufactured loop stitch for soft-tissue fixation: a biomechanical study. Arthroscopy 2010;26(12):1662–6.

30. Herzenberg JE, Lamm BM, Corwin C, et al. Isolated recession of the gastrocnemius muscle: the baumann procedure. Foot Ankle Int 2007;28(11):1154–9.

31. Abraham E, Pankovich AM. Neglected rupture of the Achilles tendon. Treatment by V-Y tendinous flap. J Bone Joint Surg Am 1975;57:253–5.

32. Nilsson-Helander K, Swärd L, Silbernagel KG, et al. A new surgical method to treat chronic ruptures and reruptures of the Achilles tendon. Knee Surg Sports Traumatol Arthr 2008;16:614.

33. Us AK, Belgin SS, Aydin T, et al. Repair of neglected Achilles tendon rupture: procedures and functional results. Arch Orthop Trauma Surg 1997;116:408–11.

34. Kissel CG, Blacklidge DK, Crowley DL. Repair of neglected Achilles ruptures: procedure and functional results. J Foot Ankle Surg 1994;33:46–52.

35. Elias I, Besser M, Nazaria LN, et al. Reconstruction for missed or neglected Achilles tendon rupture with V-Y lengthening and flexor hallucis longus tendon transfer through one incision. Foot Ankle Int 2007;28(12):1238–48.
36. Bosworth DM. Repair of defects in the tendo achillis. J Bone Joint Surg Am 1956; 38:111–4.
37. Lee YS, Lin CC, Chen CN, et al. Reconstruction for neglected Achilles tendon rupture: the modified Bosworth technique. Orthopedics 2005;28:647—50.
38. Khiami F, Di Schino M, Sariali E, et al. Treatment of chronic Achilles tendon rupture by shortening suture and free sural triceps aponeurosis graft. Orthop Traumatol Surg Res 2013;99:585—591.
39. Guclu B, Basat HC, Yildirim T, et al. Long-term results of chronic achilles tendon ruptures repaired with V-Y tendon plasty and fascia turndown. Foot Ankle Int 2016;37(7):737–42.
40. Lindholm A. A new method of operation in subcutaneous rupture of the Achilles tendon. Acta Chir Scand 1959;117:261–70.
41. Ozan F, Dogar F, Gurbuz K, et al. Chronic achilles tendon rupture reconstruction using the lindholm method and the vulpius method. J Clin Med Res 2017;9(7): 573–8.
42. Zayda AI. V-Y plasty and plantaris tendon augmentation repair in treatment of chronic ruptured achilles tendon. Biomed J Sci Tech Res 2018;2(5):2912–6.
43. Akgun U, Erol B, Karahan M. Primary surgical repair with the Krackow technique combined with plantaris tendon augmentation in the treatment of acute Achilles tendon ruptures. Acta Orthop Traumatol Turc 2006;40:228–33 [in Turkish].
44. Sadek AF, Fouly EH, Laklok MA, et al. Functional and MRI follow-up after reconstruction of chronic ruptures of the achilles tendon myerson type III using the triple-loop plantaris tendon wrapped with central turndown flap: a case series. J Orthop Surg Res 2015;10(1):109.
45. Jain P, Dutta P, Goswami P, et al. Management of neglected Achilles tendon division: assessment of two novel and innovative techniques. Adv Orthop Surg 2014;1:1–6.
46. Lin JL. Tendon transfers for achilles reconstruction. Foot Ankle Clin 2009;14(4): 729–44.
47. Nagakiran KV, Nambiar SM, Soraganvi P, et al. Flexor Hallucis Longus vs. Peroneus Brevis: the Better Tendon for Augmentation Surgery in Chronic Achilles Tendon Ruptures. Int J Res Orthopaedics 2019;5(2):264.
48. Silver RL, de la Garza J, Rang M. The myth of muscle balance. A study of relative strengths and excursions of normal muscles about the foot and ankle. J Bone Joint Surg Br 1985;67:432–7.
49. Gallant GG, Massie C, Turco VJ. Assessment of eversion and plantar flexion strength after repair of Achilles tendon rupture using peroneus brevis tendon transfer. Am J Orthop 1995;24(3):257–61.
50. Pintore E, Barra V, Pintore R, et al. Peroneus brevis tendon transfer in neglected tears of the Achilles tendon. J Trauma 2001;50:71–8.
51. Chan JY, Elliott AJ, Ellis SJ. Reconstruction of Achilles Rerupture with peroneus longus tendon transfer. Foot Ankle Int 2013;34(6):898–903.
52. Wang CC, Lin L-C, Hsu C-K, et al. Anatomic reconstruction of neglected Achilles Tendon Rupture with Autogenous Peroneal Longus Tendon by EndoButton fixation. J Trauma Inj Infect Crit Care 2009;67(5):1109–12.
53. Mann RA, Holmes GB, Seale KS, et al. Chronic rupture of the Achilles Tendon. J Bone Joint Surg 1991;73(2):214–9.

54. Lin JL. Tendon transfers for Achilles Reconstruction. Foot Ankle Clin 2009;14(4): 729–44.

55. Frenette JP, Jackson DW. Lacerations of the flexor hallucis longus in the young athlete. J Bone Joint Surg Am 1977;59(5):673–6.

56. Goss DA, Halverson A, Philbin TM, et al. Minimally invasive retrograde method of harvesting the flexor Hallucis Longus tendon: a cadaveric study. Foot Ankle Int 2019;40(10):1214–8.

57. Vega J, Vilá J, Batista J, et al. Endoscopic flexor Hallucis Longus transfer for chronic noninsertional Achilles Tendon rupture. Foot Ankle Int 2018;39(12): 1464–72.

58. Coull R, Flavin R, Stephens MM. Flexor hallucis longus transfer: evaluation of postoperative morbidity. Foot Ankle Int 2003;24(12):931–4.

59. Elias I, Raikin SM, Besser MP, et al. Outcomes of chronic insertional Achilles tendon using FHL autograft through single incision. Foot Ankle Int 2009;30(3): 199–204.

60. Wapner KL, Pavlock GS, Hecht PJ, et al. Repair of chronic Achilles tendon rupture with flexor hallucis longus tendon transfer. Foot Ankle 1993;14(8):443–9.

61. Ahmad CS, Gardner TR, Groh M, et al. Mechanical properties of soft tissue femoral fixation devices for anterior cruciate ligament reconstruction. Am J Sports Med 2004;32:635–40.

62. Sutton KM, Dodds SD, Ahmad CS, et al. Surgical treatment of distal biceps rupture. J Am Acad Orthop Surg 2010;18:139–48.

63. Mazzocca AD, Burton KJ, Romeo AA, et al. Biomechanical evaluation of 4 techniquesof distal biceps brachii tendon repair. Am J Sports Med 2007;35:252–8.

64. Wijdicks CA, Brand EJ, Nuckley DJ, et al. Biomechanical evaluation of a medial knee reconstruction with comparison of a bioabsorbable interference screw constructs and optimization with a cortical button. Knee Surg Sports Traumatol Arthrosc 2010;18:1532–41.

65. Hahn F, Meyer P, Maiwald C, et al. Treatment of chronic Achilles tendinopathy and ruptures with flexor hallucis tendon transfer: clinical outcome and MRI findings. Foot Ankle Int 2008;29(8):794–802.

66. Maffulli N, Del Buono A, Loppini M, et al. Ipsilateral free semitendinosus tendon graft with interference screw fixation for minimally invasive reconstruction of chronic tears of the Achilles tendon. Oper Orthop Traumatol 2014;26:513.

67. Patil SSD, Patil VSD, Basa VR, et al. Semitendinosus Tendon Autograft for reconstruction of large defects in chronic Achilles Tendon ruptures. Foot Ankle Int 2014;35(7):699–705.

68. Kelahmetoglu O, Gules ME, Elmadag NM, et al. Double-layer reconstruction of the Achilles' Tendon using a modified Lindholm's Technique and Vascularized Fascia Lata. J Hand Microsurg 2017;10(01):49–51. https://doi.org/10.1055/s-0037-1608745.

69. Cienfuegos A, Holgado MI, Díaz Del Río JM, et al. Chronic Achilles rupture reconstructed with Achilles tendon allograft: a case report. J Foot Ankle Surg 2013; 52(1):95–8.

70. Lepow GM, Green JB. Reconstruction of a neglected Achilles tendon rupture with an Achilles tendon allograft: a case report. J Foot Ankle Surg 2006;45(5):351–5.

71. Deese JM, Gratto-cox G, Clements FD, et al. Achilles allograft reconstruction for chronic achilles tendinopathy. J Surg Orthop Adv 2015;24(1):75–8.

72. Ofili KP, Pollard JD, Schuberth JM. The neglected Achilles tendon rupture repaired with allograft: a review of 14 cases. J Foot Ankle Surg 2016;55(6):1245–8.

Revision Surgery for Peroneal Tendon Tears

Scott C. Nelson, DPM

KEYWORDS

- Peroneal tendon tears • Revisional surgery • Tendon graft

KEY POINTS

- Peroneal tendon revision for recurrent tears requires a high level of suspicion and thorough mechanical evaluation with advanced imaging for accurate evaluation.
- Tendon degeneration is often found intraoperatively and requires tendon transfer or tendon graft to aid in restoration of mechanical strength.
- Postoperative recovery is often longer than the primary repair surgical procedures, and management of patient expectations is recommended.

INTRODUCTION

Peroneal tendons are the musculature located laterally on the lower leg, the name being derived from peroneus, or perone fibula, from the Greek peronē, to pin, and from peirein, to pierce.[1] The origin of the muscles are the proximal two-thirds of the fibula and intermuscular septa, and it inserts into the medial cuneiform/first metatarsal base (longus) and fifth metatarsal (brevis). Both the longus and brevis travel posterior to the distal fibula held within the fibular groove by the superior peroneal retinaculum.

Peroneal tendon tears are often associated with lateral ankle injuries and often lead to weakness and instability. There are several factors that can lead to progression of tendinopathy, including anatomic factors as well as factors associated with altered biomechanics. The causative factors have often been associated with lateral ankle instability, ankle sprains, ankle fractures, overuse syndromes, and calcaneal varus deformity.[2,3] The diagnosis of peroneal tendon injuries is often difficult, and it has been reported that only 60% of injuries are diagnosed on the first visit.[4] Because the peroneus brevis is located in the fibular groove posterior to the lateral malleolus and anterior to the peroneus longus tendon, it predisposes the tendon to dynamic mechanical compression and insult in the fibular groove, which may lead to tendon tears. The incidence of peroneal tendon tears was studied in cadavers by Sobel and colleagues[5] and was found to be between 11.3% and 37%.

Department of Orthopedics, Catholic Health Initiatives (CHI Health), 16909 Lakeside Hills Court Suite 208, Omaha, NE 68130, USA
E-mail address: Scn4dpm@gmail.com
Twitter: @docnelle (S.C.N.)

Clin Podiatr Med Surg 37 (2020) 569–576
https://doi.org/10.1016/j.cpm.2020.03.008
0891-8422/20/© 2020 Elsevier Inc. All rights reserved.

Surgical treatment options for peroneus tendon tears may include primary tendon repair, debridement of tendinopathy, tubularization of tendon, tenodesis/tendon transfer, excision of low-lying peroneal brevis muscle, lateral ankle ligament repair, allograft repair, peroneal groove deepening, or peroneal retinaculum repair/tightening.[6] Surgical decision making requires that the patient-specific anatomic issues and biomechanics are be taken into consideration. A good clinical examination and a high index of suspicion based on the patient's history are paramount for accurate identification. It is important to evaluate the entire lower extremity and compare the foot position and the alignment of the foot to the leg. Any subtle varus of the heel may clue the surgeon to a possible Charcot-Marie-Tooth disorder and may require additional neurologic work-up. Lateral ankle ligament integrity with stress testing and circumduction of the ankle to check for subluxation of the tendons is recommended. If less than 50% of the cross-sectional tendon is present, debridement and tubularization of the tendon is common. Greater than 50% of the cross-sectional tissue often requires tenodesis to the adjacent intact peroneal tendon if possible, or grafting when both tendons are found to be nonfunctional.[7] MRI is often required to evaluate the amount of tendon disorder present for surgical consideration, and determination allows surgical planning for possible allograft.[8]

The literature regarding revision surgery for peroneal tendon surgery is scant. When faced with a patient that has failed a primary repair, it behooves the physician to use advanced imaging and maintain a high level of suspicion if the surgical outcome is questionable and pain and weakness/instability persist. Allograft tendon seems to have a high level of success if additional tissue is needed because of degeneration.[9] The advent of biologics, including human amniotic allograft (HAA), has also assisted foot and ankle surgeons in allowing better outcomes and these should be included in the surgical plan for revision repair of peroneal tendon tears.[10] HAA has been used in several situations and is advantageous because it is immunologically inert and its high-molecular-weight hyaluronic acid reduces adhesions, fibrosis, and scar formation.

SURGICAL CONSIDERATIONS

After careful clinical and radiographic evaluation, if the decision is made to proceed with revision repair of the peroneal tendon, it is paramount that patient outcome expectations be discussed. As with any revision surgery, it is important to clearly identify factors to ensure success for the patient. In our scenario, we go over the tendon repair itself but it is important to consider ancillary procedures, including lateral ankle stabilization, calcaneal osteotomy (closing wedge), and possible fibular groove deepening depending on each individual case.

SURGICAL CASES
Case 1: Peroneal Anastomosis with Human Amniotic Allograft

A 52-year-old patient with a history of previous peroneal brevis split tear surgically repaired 14 months earlier presented with continued pain and lateral ankle weakness. MRI indicated progression of the split tear involving greater than 50% of the brevis tendon. Concomitant peroneal longus tendinosis was present and needed to be addressed.

- Standard surgical approach was from a lateral incision directed over the peroneal tendons (**Fig. 1**).

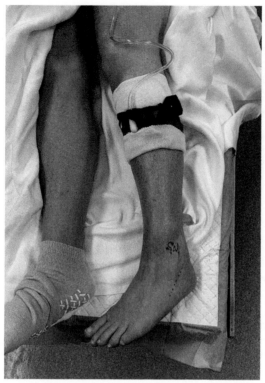

Fig. 1. Common surgical positioning is to place a lateral hip bump or bean bag to internally rotate the lower extremity for direct visualization of the lateral ankle.

- Surgical anastomosis of the peroneal brevis and longus was done with nonabsorbable #2 braided blend of polyester and polyethylene suture (**Fig. 2**).
- The repair site was wrapped with HAA (Amniofix) to augment the repair site and prevent synovial adhesions. The HAA graft was wrapped around the tendon and sutured in place with 4-0 Monocryl (poliglecaprone 25) suture (**Fig. 3**).
- The tendon sheath was closed with absorbable suture and layered skin closure performed in a standard technique. Postoperative dressings and posterior splint was applied for 2 weeks. Further immobilization was done with a pneumatic walking boot and passive range of motion was allowed at 2 weeks.
- Weight bearing was initiated at 4 weeks postoperative in a pneumatic walking boot for 4 weeks.
- Physical therapy was initiated at week 6 postoperative and activity progressed sequentially.

Case 2: Tendon Allograft with Human Amniotic Allograft

A 46-year-old woman with previous surgical anastomosis of the peroneal tendon and lateral ankle stabilization 2 years earlier. Pain and weakness persist along the lateral ankle and MRI was done to evaluate the surgical site (**Fig. 4**). MRI indicated peroneal brevis degeneration with complete rupture and peroneal longus tendinosis involving most of the tendon.

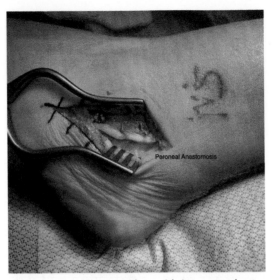

Fig. 2. Peroneal tendon anastomosis is complete with interrupted sutures.

- Surgical findings corroborated the MRI findings with complete rupture of the peroneal brevis tendon and tendinosis of the peroneal longus (**Fig. 5**).
- Surgical repair required tendon allograft to give sufficient material to reconnect the peroneal brevis tendon from its healthy portions both proximally and distally (**Fig. 6**).
- Anastomosis of the peroneal brevis and longus was done with #2 braided blend of polyester and polyethylene suture (**Fig. 7**).
- HAA (Amnion Matrix Graft) was used to prevent adhesions and aid in surgical repair. The HAA graft was wrapped around the tendon and sutured in place with 4-0 Monocryl (poliglecaprone 25) suture (**Fig. 8**).

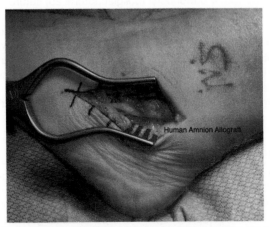

Fig. 3. HAA is applied to the surgical site to prevent adhesions and assist in surgical healing.

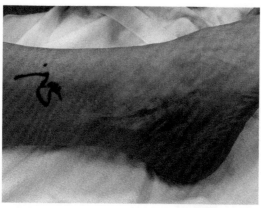

Fig. 4. Surgical scar tissue.

- The tendon sheath was closed with absorbable suture and layered skin closure performed in a standard technique. Surgical excision of scar tissue was performed and primary closure of the skin as a standard layered technique. Postoperative dressings and posterior splint were applied for 2 weeks. Continued immobilization was done with a short-leg cast for 6 weeks.
- Weight bearing was initiated at 8 weeks postoperative in a pneumatic walking boot for 4 weeks.
- Physical therapy was initiated at week 10 postoperative and activity progressed sequentially.

REHABILITATION STUDIES

In total, 49 studies were reviewed by van Dijk and colleagues[11] regarding rehabilitation of peroneal tendon repairs. No studies were found with the primary purpose to report on rehabilitation of surgically treated peroneal tendon tears or ruptures, reaffirming the

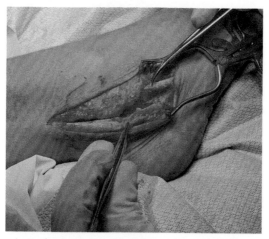

Fig. 5. Peroneal brevis tendon rupture with distal stump visualized.

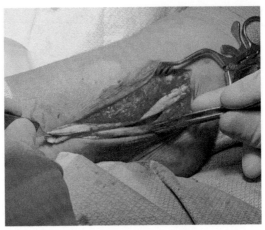

Fig. 6. Cadaveric tendon allograft used for peroneal brevis repair.

lack of scientific data for standardized treatment protocols. The results did show a median duration of the total immobilization period after primary repair of 6.0 weeks (range, 0–12 weeks), 7.0 weeks (range, 3.0–13 weeks) after tenodesis, 6.3 weeks (range, 3.0–13 weeks) after grafting, and 8.0 weeks (range, 6.0–11 weeks) after end-to-end suturing. Forty-one percent of the studies that reported on the start of range-of-motion exercises initiated range of motion within 4 weeks after surgery. No difference was found in duration of immobilization or start of range of motion between different types of surgical treatment options.

There seems to be a shift toward shorter immobilization time and early range of motion, with the understanding that there is no consensus made regarding peroneal revision repair. It is more important to adjust the rehabilitation protocol to every specific patient for optimal rehabilitation and recovery.

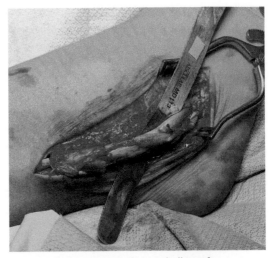

Fig. 7. Anastomosis of peroneal longus tendon and allograft.

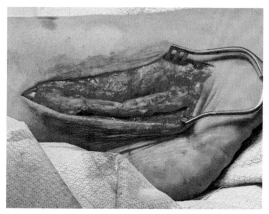

Fig. 8. HAA applied to surgical repair site to prevent tenosynovial adhesions.

SUMMARY

Peroneal tendon revision surgery has little literature regarding surgical treatment outcomes and postoperative recovery protocols. It behooves foot and ankle surgeons to consider all options for repair, take into account the mechanical reasons why the original surgery failed, and address those issues to optimize successful outcome. Significant tendon degeneration may be present and can be identified preoperatively with MRI. If there is significant degeneration (>50%), then tendon allograft is strongly recommended. It is important to educate patients on realistic outcomes and also expected goals. The postoperative recovery is variable and is often based on ancillary procedures, but early active range of motion should be initiated as soon as possible to avoid adhesion issues. Additional advances with human amniotic membrane allografts to prevent synovial tendon adhesions can help ensure optimized outcomes for revision peroneal tendon surgical repairs.

DISCLOSURE

The authors have nothing to disclose.

REFERENCES

1. "Peroneal." The Merriam-Webster.com dictionary, Merriam-Webster Inc. Available at: https://www.merriam-webster.com/dictionary/peroneal. Accessed February 20, 2020.
2. Clarke HD, Kitaoka HB, Ehman RL. Peroneal tendon injuries. Foot Ankle Int 1998; 19(5):280–8.
3. Krause JO, Brodsky JW. Peroneus brevis tendon tears: pathophysiology, surgical reconstruction and clinical results. Foot Ankle Int 1998;19(5):271–9.
4. Dombek MF, Lamm BM, Saltrick K, et al. Peroneal tendon tears: a retrospective review. J Foot Ankle Surg 2003;42(5):250–8.
5. Sobel M, Bohne WHO, DiCarlo E, et al. Longitudinal splitting of the peroneus brevis tendon: an anatomic and histologic study of cadaveric material. Foot Ankle 1991;12:165–70.
6. Heckman DS, Reddy S, Pedowitz D, et al. Operative treatment for peroneal tendon disorders. J Bone Joint Surg Am 2008;90(2):404–18.

7. Redfern D, Myerson M. The management of concomitant tears of the peroneus longus and brevis tendons. Foot Ankle Int 2004;25:695–707.

8. Lamm BM, Myers DT, Dombek M, et al. Magnetic resonance imaging and surgical correlation of peroneus brevis tears. J Foot Ankle Surg 2004;43(1):30–6.

9. Mook WR, Parekh SG, Nunley JA. Allograft reconstruction of peroneal tendons: operative technique and clinical outcomes. Foot Ankle Int 2013;34(9):1212–20.

10. Anderson JJ, Adeleke T, Rice BB, et al. Surgical treatment of peroneus brevis tendon repair with and without human amniotic allograft: a comparison study. Knee Surg Sports Traumatol Arthrosc 2016;24:1165–74.

11. van Dijk PA, Lubberts B, Verheul C, et al. Rehabilitation after surgical treatment of peroneal tendon tears and ruptures. Knee Surg Sports Traumatol Arthrosc 2016; 24(4):1165–74.

Revision of the Chronic Syndesmotic Injury

Sean T. Grambart, DPM[a,b],*, Ryan D. Prusa, DPM, PGY1[b], Katherine M. Ternent, BA[a]

KEYWORDS

- Syndesmosis • Ankle fracture • Chronic syndesmotic injury • Malreduction

KEY POINTS

- Failed anatomic reduction of the syndesmosis can lead to chronic pain and limitations.
- Complete evaluation of the fracture including thorough evaluation of the posterior malleolar fragment can aid in the diagnosis and reduction of syndesmotic injuries.
- Reconstruction of a chronic, malreduced syndesmosis can lead to improved functional outcome and decrease pain.

ANATOMY AND BIOMECHANICS OF THE SYNDESMOSIS

There is a great deal of variety between individuals when discussing the anatomy of the syndesmosis.[1–5] However, within the specific individual, there is minimal difference between the right and left lower extremity. Dikos and colleagues[6] computed tomography (CT) evaluation showed no more than 2.3-mm difference of the tibiofibular interval within individuals. Within the overall joint structure, the incisura plays an important role in stability. In most people, the fibula is positioned along the central or anterior portion of the incisura. The larger anterior tubercle prevents the forward translation of the fibula along the talus.[7] Boszczyk and colleagues[5] evaluated the incisura in detail in regard to reduction. The results of their study indicate that certain morphologic configurations of the tibial incisura increased the risk of specific syndesmotic malreduction patterns. Anteversion of the incisura correlated with anterior displacement of the fibula, whereas retroversion of the incisura correlated with posterior fibular displacement. They also showed that deep and disengaged syndesmosis were more prone to overcompression.

The syndesmosis ligamentous area is formed by four fibrous structures: (1) the anterior inferior tibiofibular ligament (AITFL), (2) posterior inferior tibiofibular ligament

[a] Des Moines University, College of Podiatric Medicine and Surgery, 3200 Grand Avenue, Des Moines, IA 50312, USA; [b] Unitypoint Health - Iowa Methodist Medical Center, 1200 Pleasant Street, Des Moines, IA 50309, USA
* Corresponding author. Des Moines University, College of Podiatric Medicine and Surgery, 3200 Grand Avenue, Des Moines, IA 50312.
E-mail address: Sean.Grambart@dmu.edu

Clin Podiatr Med Surg 37 (2020) 577–592
https://doi.org/10.1016/j.cpm.2020.03.011
podiatric.theclinics.com

(PITFL), (3) transverse ligament, and (4) the tibiofibular interosseous membrane.[8] The AITFL originates from the anterior-lateral tubercle of the tibia and extends inferiorly and attaches at the anterior border of the lateral malleolus. Sometimes the PITFL is divided into the superficial and deep. The deep component is more commonly referred to the deep transverse ligament. The PITFL extends obliquely from the lateral malleolus to a broad attachment on the posterolateral tibia tubercle. The transverse ligament is thick and strong and originates from the round posterior fibular tubercle, inserting on the lower part of the posterior border of the tibial articular surface. This deep portion is more transverse and acts as a labrum, deepening the tibial articular surface. Finally, the interosseous membrane spans most of the length of the lower leg between the tibia and fibula. The ligament begins along the proximal tibiofibular junction and extends distally to terminate just superior to the AITFL and PITFL.[4,9–15]

Biomechanically, the normal ankle joint with an intact syndesmosis prevents lateral fibular translation during weightbearing, enabling the fibula to bear 10% to 17% of the weightbearing load during gait.[16] With normal mechanics, the ankle does require some translation and rotation of the fibula. With dorsiflexion there is an average of 2.5° of external rotation of the fibula, whereas plantarflexion results in less than 1° of internal rotation.[17] In normal individuals, external rotation force causes external rotation, medial translation, and posterior displacement of the fibula through the syndesmosis.[18] These syndesmotic ligaments mainly stabilize and prevent lateral fibular translation during weightloading ambulation. Each of these ligaments provides a different amount of stability from one another: the AITFL provides 35%, the transverse ligament gives 33%, tibiofibular interosseous membrane gives 22%, and the PITFL gives 9%.[19] The peroneal artery and its branches are the main blood supply of the syndesmosis. The interosseous ligament is perforated by the artery 3 cm proximal to the ankle joint, so it is at a greater risk of slow healing because of a syndesmotic vascular insult.[20]

CHRONIC SYNDESMOTIC INJURIES

Chronic syndesmotic pathology is usually a result of a missed diagnosis, malunion of an ankle fracture, malreduction at the time of fixation, or failure of fixation before complete healing of the syndesmosis. With sprains and fractures around the ankle, the physician can fail to diagnose or appreciate the extent of the syndesmotic injury and subsequently fail to fixate it correctly.[21] This can cause slow healing and longer periods of pain in the area. Syndesmotic injuries can occur in 18% of ankle sprains but that chance increases up to 32% in athletes.[22,23] They usually occur with external rotation accompanied by plantarflexion or dorsiflexion. In sports, these movements can happen when planting the foot and then quickly changing directions.[23]

With ankle fracture, historical belief is that syndesmotic injuries occur when fracture of the lateral malleolus starts above the ankle joint, such as in the case of a pronation-external rotation injury or Weber C (Wb C) ankle fracture. Chun and colleagues[24] investigated preoperative detection of syndesmotic injury according to fracture patterns in supination external rotation (SER) III and IV ankle fractures by using radiography and CT. All SER III and IV ankle fracture were retrospectively reviewed. A total of 52 patients with SER III, 75 patients with SER IV, and 27 patients with SER IV equivalent ankle fractures were identified. Almost 70% showed injury and instability of the syndesmosis. The cutoff values of these factors were 4.4 mm and 32.8°, respectively. They concluded that CT was superior to simple radiography in predicting syndesmotic injury at the preoperative period in SER III and IV. Medial space widening and fragment angle of the fibular posterior cortex, as predictive factors, showed significant correlations. Shelton and colleagues[21] suggest that all Wb C fractures, and any Wb B fracture in which full surgical reduction is questionable, should be checked with a CT scan for a syndesmotic injury. Therefore, the surgeon should have a high suspicion for syndesmotic injury with pronation external rotation fractures and SER fracture patterns including proximal fibular fractures.[15,23,24]

MALREDUCTION OF THE SYNDESMOSIS

It is unknown what the overall rate of syndesmotic malreduction is; it is just known that they are a complication of ankle fracture surgeries. This is a result of inadequate reduction the fracture and syndesmosis or failure to recognize a syndesmotic injury. Gardner and colleagues[25] conducted a study with a cohort of 25 patients, and found 13 (52%) of the patients to have a surgically malreduced syndesmosis. Shelton and colleagues[21] studied 187 subjects with ankle fractures and found that 44 (23.6%) had malreduced syndesmosis.

Mason and coworkers[26] studied the posterior malleolus fracture extensively in their 2017 study with proposed classification system. They found that the primary posterior malleolar fracture fragments were characterized into three groups. Type 1 fracture was described as a small extra-articular posterior malleolar primary fragment. Type 2 fractures consisted of a primary fragment of the posterolateral triangle of the tibia. Type 3 primary fragment was characterized by a coronal plane fracture line involving the whole posterior plafond. Syndesmotic injuries were present in 100% of type 1 fractures. In type 2 posterior malleolar fractures, there was a variable medial injury with mixed avulsion/impaction cause. In type 3 posterior malleolar fractures, most fibular fractures were either a high fracture or a long oblique fracture in the same fracture alignment as the posterior shear tibia fragment. Most medial injuries were Y-type or posterior oblique fractures. This fracture pattern had a low incidence of syndesmotic injury.

Imaging is used intraoperatively or postoperatively to view if the syndesmosis has been properly reduced. The most common and accessible are intraoperative radiographs, but postoperative CT scans have been found to be the most reliable at identifying a malreduced syndesmosis. However, at the time of the postoperative CT, if the syndesmosis is found to be malreduced, the surgeon would have to wait and go back in for a revisional syndesmotic surgery.[27] Intraoperative radiographs are taken of the ankle to look at the tibiofibular relationship right away. The best views to see the important structures on radiograph would be anterior-posterior (AP) ankle, mortise ankle, and lateral ankle. With these views the observer can look at the AP tibiofibular clear space (normal is <6 mm), AP tibiofibular overlap (normal is >6 mm), mortise tibiofibular overlap (normal is >1 mm), and mortise medial clear space (normal is <5 mm).[25,28] If the radiographs come back inconclusive, then external rotation stress testing mortise radiographs are obtained.[23,29] Plain films are not always accurate because it is difficult to assess the syndesmotic congruency.[21] Thus, axial CT scans are taken 1 cm proximal to the ankle joint to measure the distance between the anterior and posterior lateral tibial tubercles to the fibula. These anterior and posterior tubercle distances for a fully reduced syndesmosis should be within 1 mm of each other. If they are not, there could be fibular rotation, fibular displacement, or decreased fibular length present.[15,25,28] These measurements are not based on evidence-based numbers, however, because each patient's anatomy is different. Thus, the injured ankle should be confirmed with imaging of the patient's own contralateral uninjured ankle.[30] MRI is used to view the soft tissue to confirm a malre-duction, which can present as hypertrophic syndesmotic ligaments. Arthroscopy is another method that allows the surgeon to directly visualize the syndesmotic struc-tures. With arthroscopy, the diagnosis of a malreduced syndesmosis is based on the presence of hypermobility between the tibia and fibula and identifying hypertrophic syndesmosis ligaments. Arthroscopy is also used for the management of a chronic malreduced syndesmosis by correcting intra-articular pathology that forms because of the anatomic instability.[29]

Chronic malreduced syndesmotic injuries can cause further problems in the ankle, such as osteoarthritis. Other symptoms include chronic pain, swelling, popping, insta-bility, stiffness, and limited dorsiflexion.[16,31] From a functional standpoint, Sagi and colleagues[32] retrospectively reviewed 107 ankle fractures with associated syndes-motic injuries requiring reduction and fixation. All patients were evaluated at a mini-mum of 2 years follow-up with 68 patients available for follow-up. Fifteen percent of the open syndesmotic reductions were malreduced on postoperative CT scans, whereas 44% of the closed syndesmotic reductions were malreduced on postopera-tive CT scan. Patients with a malreduced syndesmosis recorded significantly worse functional outcome scores. The authors recommended that surgeons not only perform a direct, open visualization of the syndesmosis during the reduction maneuver, but obtain a postoperative CT scan with comparison to the contralateral extremity as well.

With the patient's symptoms, the goal should be getting the patient back to optimal functioning, alignment, and minimizing pain. Harper[31] studied six patients who had pain, swelling, and popping from a malreduced syndesmosis. The average amount of time for each of the patients postreduction of their syndesmosis was 15 months. After the surgical correction, five of the six patients were absent of joint widening, pain, and instability at the 2-year mark. With the results, expectations are in patients with chronic injury and scarring from a malreduced syndesmosis, late reconstruction can lead to improvement in their symptoms. In a case study by Beals and Manoli,[33] 2 months after a failed surgical syndesmotic reduction, the patient had an American Orthopaedic Foot and Ankle Society (AOFAS) score of 67. At 26 months after second syndesmotic reduction surgery, AOFAS score was 100.

A technique involved osteotomizing and mobilizing the insertion of the AITFL with a 1 × 1 cm bone block. After application of maximal compression to the mortise with a pelvic clamp, the bone block was advanced into the gutter and stabilized with screw fix-ation. The bone block was supplemented with a tetracortical syndesmotic screw. Follow-up demonstrated improved average AOFAS scores (75–92) in 12 patients treated greater than 2 years after initial injury with an average follow-up of 25 months.[34]

Allograft reconstruction has been performed with good results. Grass and col-leagues[35] used a split peroneus longus tendon autograft with a tricortical transfix-ation screw in a series of 16 patients. At an average follow-up of 16 months, 15 of 16 patients reported pain relief and stated they would undergo the surgery again. Morris and colleagues[36] used hamstring allograft anatomically to reconstruct the AITFL and the interosseous ligament using two tunnels. The graft was then passed medial to lateral through tunnel one and finally looped over the fibula into tunnel two. The graft was secured medially and laterally with 15-mm interference screws. Visual analog pain scores improved and the average postoperative AOFAS score was 85.4. The graft used in this technique was 7 to 8 mm in diameter compared with the previously described peroneus graft, which was only 3.5 mm in diameter.

In a recent systematic literature review, 17 retrospective or prospective case series showed good functional outcomes and low complication rates were reported.[37] The authors concluded that with the few studies that have reported there are several different techniques used to treat this problem. They stated that quality of current studies is overall satisfactory but could be improved with larger patient numbers and prospective analysis. Recognition of this clinical entity as an identifiable and treatable cause of ankle pain requires vigilant clinical investigation. With evaluation of all of the present studies, this can lead us to believe that after the syndesmosis was fully reduced, the joint was able to revert to improved function with improvement of clinical symptoms.

SURGICAL TECHNIQUE

This is a 39-year-old man with history of a Wb C bimalleolar ankle variant ankle injury. Open reduction/internal fixation was performed. The patient presented to the primary

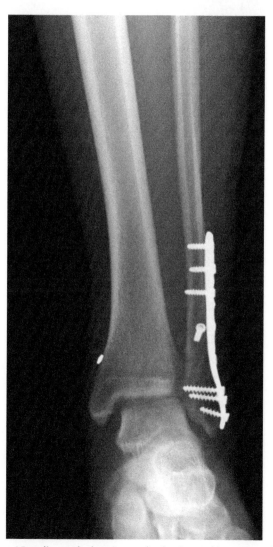

Fig. 1. Preoperative AP radiograph showing malreduction ankle and syndesmosis.

author's office (STG) approximately 12 months after the initial surgery with complaints of worsening pain in the ankle and limitations with activities. Radiographs and MRI show instability with malreduction of the syndesmosis (**Figs. 1–3**). Conservative treatment with therapy and bracing was unsuccessful and patient elected to perform revision.

The patient is positioned supine on the operating room table. A bump is placed under the ipsilateral hip to help expose the lateral ankle. If ankle arthroscopy is performed, the bump may be placed after the arthroscopy is complete. A thigh tourniquet is applied. The leg is prepared and draped to make sure the knee is visible to serve as a reference point if needed.

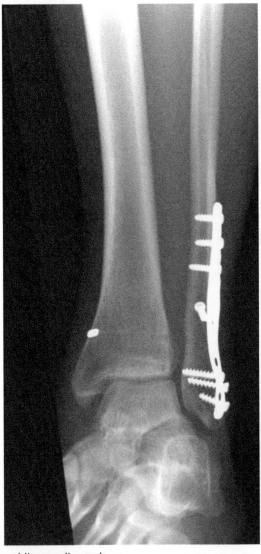

Fig. 2. Preoperative oblique radiograph.

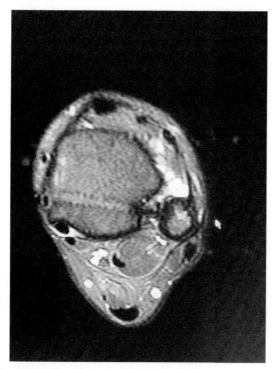

Fig. 3. Preoperative MRI with widening of the syndesmosis.

Arthroscopic procedures are performed before the syndesmotic reconstruction. A linear incision is made along the distal fibula. This incision is placed slightly more anterior to midline of the fibula and can extend distally toward the lateral ankle joint line.

The incision is deepened with care to protect the intermediate dorsal cutaneous branch off of the superficial peroneal nerve and the deep peroneal artery. This typically is retracted medially with minimal tension on the nerve. As the dissection is deepened, the peroneal tendons is exposed and inspected for any damage. By

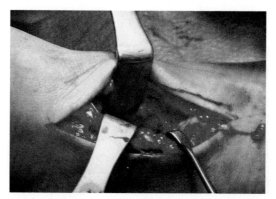

Fig. 4. Anterior-lateral ankle exposure that can help facilitate reduction.

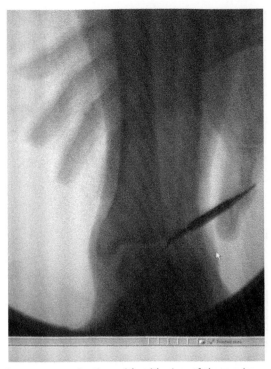

Fig. 5. Intraoperative stress examination with widening of the syndesmosis.

exposing the lateral ankle joint this can help aid in accurately reducing the syndesmosis (**Fig. 4**). Hardware along the fibula is removed at this time. Once the hardware is removed, intraoperative stress examination shows the chronic instability of the syndesmosis (**Fig. 5**). There is normally a significant amount of scar tissue within the syndesmosis that needs to be removed to allow for reduction (**Fig. 6**). Care must be taken to avoid injury to the peroneal artery, which can be bound up in this scar tissue.

Once the syndesmosis area has been adequately prepared, the osseous tunnels are created before reduction (**Fig. 7**). This helps with the visualization of the proper

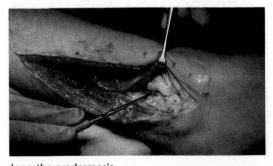

Fig. 6. Scar tissue along the syndesmosis.

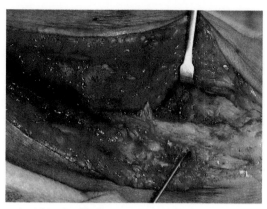

Fig. 7. Osseous tunnel within the fibula.

location of the osseous tunnel, especially the center aspect of the tibia. There are multiple ways for fixation of the syndesmosis including plate and screws, allograft, suture bracing, or a combination of the three. Allograft is preferred if there is a large amount of scar tissue that needs to be resected that leaves minimal ligamentous tissue. This is normally seen in cases in which a few years have passed between the time of the initial injury and the surgery. In cases where the malreduction is treated within a year after the initial time of injury, the ligamentous tissue seems to be better organized, which allows a type of internal suture brace. Regardless of either allograft or internal suture bracing, we do use plate and screws to help hold the reduction as the tissue heals.

We prefer to use a peroneus longus allograft because this graft is readily available, has enough length, and it gives the surgeon the option of either a round end or a flat end. The graft is thawed in warm sterile saline for approximately 10 minutes. The authors have not found the need to prestretch the graft before insertion. The graft is then cut at the junction of the flat and the circular end to separate the two. The circular side is the one that is used most of the time.

An osseous tunnel is created from the fibula into the tibia at the level of the syndesmosis (see **Fig. 7**). Once the osteotomy has been placed, the allograft is passed from the fibula into the tibia and secured into the tibia (**Fig. 8**). With chronic syndesmotic injuries with malreduction, the use of large bone clamps may be required to

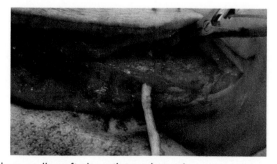

Fig. 8. Peroneus longus allograft along the syndesmosis.

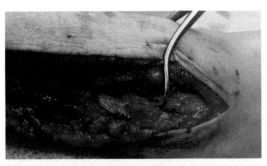

Fig. 9. Reduction of the syndesmosis with bone clamp.

help hold the reduction (**Fig. 9**). The authors prefer to use the junction of the fibula, tibia, and talus at the ankle level to check the reduction intraoperatively. The three bones should come together at a center point along the ankle. Be careful not to mistake reduction with internal rotation of the fibula, which could open the syndesmosis posteriorly leading to continued malreduction. The fibula should be reduced as a medial translation toward the tibia. After the reduction is reduced clinically, the reduction is then confirmed radiographically by checking the AP, mortise, and lateral views intraoperatively. The allograft is then secured into place along the fibula and plate fixation is often performed to help with stabilization with the soft tissue healing (**Figs. 10** and **11**).

The incision is irrigated, and layered closure is performed. After skin closure, the foot and leg is placed in a postoperative sprint with the foot and ankle in neutral position. Postoperative recovery is normally 2 weeks nonweightbearing in a splint followed by 2 weeks in a nonweightbearing cast as tolerated. At 4 weeks postoperative, the patient is advanced into a weightbearing boot. The boot is removed when sitting or sleeping but an ankle brace is applied to avoid excessive inversion and eversion. The patient can start to wean out of the boot using the ankle brace at 6 weeks postoperative. Physical therapy is typically started to assist the patient with slowly advancing activities and weaning out of the brace with walking. Normally recovery takes approximately 4 to 6 months.

In cases where there is malunion of the fibula, a derotational osteotomy or lengthening osteotomy needs to be performed. A 48-year-old man with a history

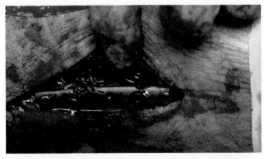

Fig. 10. Plate fixation of the fibula to aid in stability of the syndesmotic reduction.

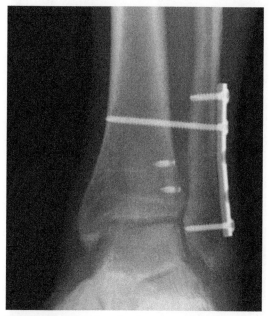

Fig. 11. Postoperative radiograph with reduction.

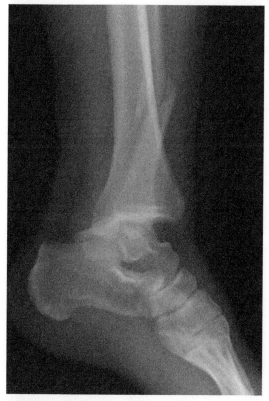

Fig. 12. Lateral ankle injury radiograph.

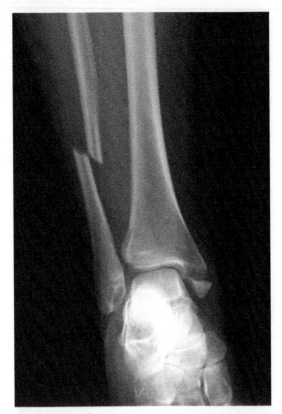

Fig. 13. AP ankle injury radiograph.

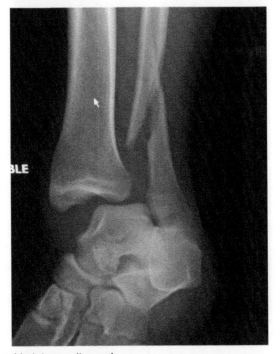

Fig. 14. Oblique ankle injury radiograph.

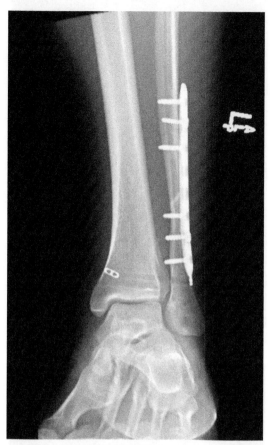

Fig. 15. AP radiograph showing malunion of fibula.

of a Wb C bimalleolar ankle fracture is shown in **Figs. 12–14**. Open reduction/internal fixation with syndesmotic fixation with internal suture bracing was performed. The patient was referred to the author's (STG) office for continued pain and limitation with activities. Radiographs and CT imaging shows malreduction of the fracture with external rotation and shortening of the fibula and malreduction of the syndesmosis (**Figs. 15** and **16**). An allograft lengthening osteotomy of the fibula was performed. Once the osteotomy is performed, the fibula is distracted out to the desired length and rotated as needed and the structural allograft is placed (**Fig. 17**). Plate fixation is performed, and the allograft syndesmotic reconstruction is performed (**Fig. 18**).

In the case of fibular lengthening, postoperative recovery is normally 2 weeks nonweightbearing in a splint followed by 4 weeks in a nonweightbearing cast as tolerated. At 6 weeks postoperative, the patient is advanced into a weightbearing boot if there is radiographic healing at the bone grafting site. The boot is removed when sitting or sleeping. The patient can start to wean out of the boot using an ankle brace at 10 weeks postoperative. Physical therapy is typically started to assist the patient with slowly advancing activities and weaning out of the brace with walking. Typical recovery takes approximately 9 to 12 months.

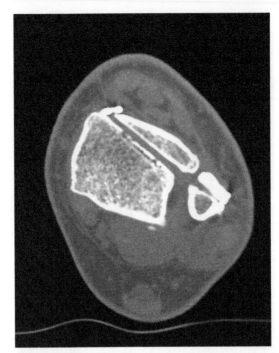

Fig. 16. Axial CT scan with malreduction of the syndesmosis.

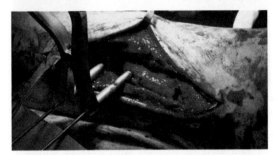

Fig. 17. Distraction osteotomy of the fibula.

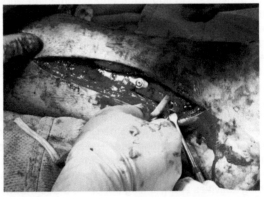

Fig. 18. Plate fixation of the distraction osteotomy with peroneal allograft for the syndesmosis.

DISCLOSURE

S.T. Grambart is a partner at BESPA Global. No conflicts with the material within this article.

REFERENCES

1. Ebraheim NA, Lu J, Yang H, et al. The fibular incisure of the tibia on CT scan: a cadaver study. Foot Ankle Int 1998;19(5):318–21.
2. Chen Y, Qiang M, Zhang K, et al. A reliable radiographic measurement for evaluation of normal distal tibiofibular syndesmosis: a multi-detector computed tomography study in adults. J Foot Ankle Res 2015;8:32.
3. Elgafy H, Semaan HB, Blessinger B, et al. Computed tomography of normal distal tibiofibular syndesmosis. Skeletal Radiol 2010;39(6):559–64.
4. Mendelsohn ES, Hoshino CM, Harris TG, et al. CT characterizing the anatomy of uninjured ankle syndesmosis. Orthopedics 2014;37(2):e157–60.
5. Boszczyk A, Kwapisz S, Krummel M, et al. Correlation of incisura anatomy with syndesmotic malreduction. Foot Ankle Int 2018;39(3):369–75.
6. Dikos GD, Heisler J, Choplin RH, et al. Normal tibiofibular relationships at the syndesmosis on axial CT imaging. J Orthop Trauma 2012;26(7):433–8.
7. Lepojarvi S, Pakarinen H, Savola O. Posterior translation of the fibula may indicate malreduction: CT study of normal variation in uninjured ankles. J Orthop Trauma 2014;28:205–9.
8. Fort NM, Aiyer AA, Kaplan JR, et al. Management of acute injuries of the tibiofibular syndesmosis. Eur J Orthop Surg Traumatol 2017;27(4):449–59.
9. Carto C, Lezak B, Varacallo M. Anatomy, Bony pelvis and lower limb, distal tibiofibular joint (tibiofibular syndesmosis) [Updated 2019 Sep 18]. In: StatPearls [Internet]. Treasure Island (FL): StatPearls Publishing; 2020.
10. Yuen CP, Lui TH. Distal tibiofibular syndesmosis: anatomy, biomechanics, injury and management. Open Orthop J 2017;11:670–7.
11. Hermans JJ, Beumer A, de Jong TA, et al. Anatomy of the distal tibiofibular syndesmosis in adults: a pictorial essay with a multimodality approach. J Anat 2010; 217(6):633–45.
12. Nault ML, Marien M, Hebert-Davies J, et al. MRI quantification of the impact of ankle position on syndesmosis anatomy. Foot Ankle Int 2017;38(2):215–9.
13. Lin CF, Gross ML, Weinhold P. Ankle syndesmosis injuries: anatomy, biomechanics, mechanism of injury, and clinical guidelines for diagnosis and intervention. J Orthop Sports Phys Ther 2006;36(6):372–84.
14. Ostrum RF, De Meo P, Subramanian R. A critical analysis of the anterior-posterior radiographic anatomy of the ankle syndesmosis. Foot Ankle Int 1995;16(3): 128–31.
15. Switaj PJ, Mendoza M, Kadakia AR. Acute and chronic injuries to the syndesmosis. Clin Sports Med 2015;34(4):643–77.
16. Espinosa N, Smerek JP, Myerson MS. Acute and chronic syndesmosis injuries: pathomechanisms, diagnosis and management. Foot Ankle Clin 2006;11(3): 639–57.
17. Michelson JD, Helgemo SL Jr. Kinematics of the axially loaded ankle. Foot Ankle Int 1995;16(9):577–82.
18. Beumer A, Valstar ER, Garling EH, et al. Kinematics of the distal tibiofibular syndesmosis: radiostereometry in 11 normal ankles. Acta Orthop Scand 2003;74(3): 337–43.

19. Ogilvie-Harris DJ, Reed SC, Hedman TP. Disruption of the ankle syndesmosis: biomechanical study of the ligamentous restraints. Arthroscopy 1994;10(5): 558–60.
20. McKeon KE, Wright RW, Johnson JE, et al. Vascular anatomy of the tibiofibular syndesmosis. J Bone Joint Surg Am 2012;94(10):931–8.
21. Shelton J, Dorman S, Doorgakant A, et al. How well do we reduce ankle fractures intra-operatively: a retrospective 1 year review using Pettrone's criteria. Foot (Edinb) 2019;40:46–53.
22. Waterman BR, Belmont PJ Jr, Cameron KL, et al. Risk factors for syndesmotic and medial ankle sprain: role of sex, sport, and level of competition. Am J Sports Med 2011;39(5):992–8.
23. Porter DA, Jaggers RR, Barnes AF, et al. Optimal management of ankle syndesmosis injuries. Open Access J Sports Med 2014;5:173–82.
24. Chun DI, Kim J, Kim YS, et al. Relationship between fracture morphology of lateral malleolus and syndesmotic stability after supination-external rotation type ankle fractures. Injury 2019;50(7):1382–7.
25. Gardner MJ, Demetrakopoulos D, Briggs SM, et al. Malreduction of the tibiofibular syndesmosis in ankle fractures. Foot Ankle Int 2006;27(10):788–92.
26. Mason LW, Marlow WJ, Widnall J, et al. Pathoanatomy and associated injuries of posterior malleolus fracture of the ankle. Foot Ankle Int 2017;38(11):1229–35.
27. van den Heuvel SB, Dingemans SA, Gardenbroek TJ, et al. Assessing quality of syndesmotic reduction in surgically treated acute syndesmotic injuries: a systematic review. J Foot Ankle Surg 2019;58(1):144–50.
28. Gardner R, Yousri T, Holmes F, et al. Stabilization of the syndesmosis in the Maisonneuve fracture: a biomechanical study comparing 2-hole locking plate and quadricortical screw fixation. J Orthop Trauma 2013;27(4):212–6.
29. Zamzami MM, Zamzam MM. Chronic isolated distal tibiofibular syndesmotic disruption: diagnosis and management. Foot Ankle Surg 2009;15(1):14–9.
30. Lilyquist M, Shaw A, Latz K, et al. Cadaveric analysis of the distal tibiofibular syndesmosis. Foot Ankle Int 2016;37(8):882–90.
31. Harper MC. Delayed reduction and stabilization of the tibiofibular syndesmosis. Foot Ankle Int 2001;22(1):15–8.
32. Sagi HC, Shah AR, Sanders RW. The functional consequence of syndesmotic joint malreduction at a minimum 2-year follow-up. J Orthop Trauma 2012;26(7): 439–43.
33. Beals TC, Manoli A 2nd. Late syndesmosis reconstruction: a case report. Foot Ankle Int 1998;19(7):485–8.
34. Wagener ML, Beumer A, Swierstra BA. Chronic instability of the anterior tibiofibular syndesmosis of the ankle. Arthroscopic findings and results of anatomical reconstruction. BMC Musculoskelet Disord 2011;12:212.
35. Grass R, Rammelt S, Biewener A, et al. Peroneus longus ligamentoplasty for chronic instability of the distal tibiofibular syndesmosis. Foot Ankle Int 2003; 24(5):392–7.
36. Morris MW, Rice P, Schneider TE. Distal tibiofibular syndesmosis reconstruction using a free hamstring autograft. Foot Ankle Int 2009;30(6):506–11.
37. Krahenbuhl N, Weinberg MW, Hintermann B, et al. Surgical outcome in chronic syndesmotic injury: a systematic literature review. Foot Ankle Surg 2019;25(5): 691–7.

Bone Grafting Options

Sean T. Grambart, DPM[a,b],*, Danika S. Anderson, BS[a],
Travis Drew Anderson, BS[a]

KEYWORDS

- Bone graft • Bone marrow aspirate allograft • Revision surgery

KEY POINTS

- Autologous bone graft has multiple harvest sites that can aid in revision surgery.
- Bone marrow aspirate offers the potential of undifferentiated mesenchymal cells.
- Allograft options are available for surgery.

AUTOLOGOUS BONE GRAFT

The so-called diamond concept of fracture healing described by Giannnoudis and colleagues[1] is based on combining osteogenic cells, osteoinductive growth factors, osteoconductive scaffolding, and the stability of the fracture to promote an optimal environment for fracture healing. Osteoinduction is a process in which new bone is formed with the use of growth factors to stimulate undifferentiated mesenchymal cells to form osteoblasts. These growth factors include bone morphogenetic protein, platelet-derived growth factor, and vascular endothelial growth factor.[2–4] Osteoconduction is the use of a scaffolding to allow the host bone, graft, and vasculature to promote healing. Osteoconductive graft properties are closely related to cancellous bone.[4] The advancements that have recently been seen in orthobiologics have been within the property of osteogenesis or the process of producing new bone. These advancements have come from the use of growth factors, cell signaling proteins, and cell-based therapies.[5]

Autologous bone graft is still the gold standard that all orthobiologics are compared with. Autologous grafts offer all of the properties mentioned earlier for the optimal bone graft, which makes them reliable when it comes to stability and optimizing the healing environment. In addition, autologous grafts also involve no risk of disease transmission to the host and are biocompatible.[6–9]

Autologous cortical bone graft is best used for defects in which mechanical stability is needed immediately. Although this type of graft provides all 3 properties, it has

[a] Des Moines University, College of Podiatric Medicine and Surgery, 3200 Grand Avenue, Des Moines, IA 50312, USA; [b] Unitypoint Health - Iowa Methodist Medical Center, 1200 Pleasant Street, Des Moines, IA 50309, USA
* Corresponding author. Des Moines University, College of Podiatric Medicine and Surgery, 3200 Grand Avenue, Des Moines, IA 50312.
E-mail address: Sean.Grambart@dmu.edu

Clin Podiatr Med Surg 37 (2020) 593–600
https://doi.org/10.1016/j.cpm.2020.03.012
0891-8422/20/© 2020 Elsevier Inc. All rights reserved.
podiatric.theclinics.com

minimal osteogenic and osteoinductive properties compared with its excellent osteo-conductive property. Vascular ingrowth is slow with cortical grafts and the healing process involves resorption for graft healing, which means the grafts become weaker over the first 6 months and then gain strength by 12 months after implantation.[9–14]

Autologous cancellous bone graft with its trabeculae lined with active osteoblasts is highly osteogenic and hence is the most common autologous bone graft.[9,13] The other advantage of the trabecular pattern is the large surface area, which de-creases the time for graft incorporation and remodeling. Studies have shown that vascularization can occur within the first 2 days after implantation, new bone forma-tion in the first couple of weeks, and remodeling at approximately 8 weeks through the process of creeping substitution when osteoblasts deposit new bone as osteo-clasts resorb necrotic donor bone at the same time.[5,10,13–15] Although this rapid turnover is ideal, it comes at the sacrifice of cancellous grafts not being inherently structurally stable.[7,9,10,14–20]

Corticocancellous grafts offer the advantages of both, and the most common loca-tion is the iliac crest. There are some disadvantages with autologous grafts, especially iliac crest, such as donor site complications (pain, infection, and limitation of quantity of graft).[10,21–23] Minimizing these potential complications from the harvest site is key when choosing locations for harvest around the foot and ankle. The quality of the graft harvested is also an important consideration. Chiodo and colleagues[24] found through histologic studies that only iliac crest contained active hematopoietic cells compared with tibial grafts, which were found to have quiescent fat and little hematopoietic marrow.

When considering the necessity of autologous graft, this requires answering a few questions[25]:

- Is autograft required?
- How much graft is needed?
- Is structural graft needed?
- Is enhanced biology needed, which may need iliac crest?

The most common locations for autologous bone grafts sites are calcaneus and the distal tibia, especially if a combination of cortical and cancellous bone is required. The distal tibia is easily accessible and offers both cortical and cancellous bone options, and has the advantages of minimal blood loss and not having a sig-nificant increase in operating room times.[19,26] A linear incision is made along the medial distal tibia taking care to stay proximal to the ankle joint and carefully retracting the saphenous nerve and vein. The periosteum is incised but not re-flected. Predrilling the area is beneficial to raise the cortical window. Rounding cor-ners can minimize the risk of stress fractures. If only cancellous bone is needed, then the cortical window can be raised with a hinge and then replaced after a curette is used to harvest cancellous bone. If cortical bone is indicated, then the cortex window can be used as well. Cancellous allografts chips can be used to fill the harvest site (**Fig. 1**).

Calcaneal autologous graft can be obtained through a lateral incision along the pos-terior aspect of the calcaneus (**Fig. 2**). The sural nerve should be anterior to the incision but care should be taken in cases of aberrant anatomy. The periosteum is raised and the graft can be harvested between the Achilles insertion site and posterior aspect of the posterior facet of the subtalar joint. The corners of the graft can be predrilled. The graft that is harvested can be a corticocancellous graft or cancellous graft (**Fig. 3**). Regardless, back-filling the harvest site with either cancellous bone chips or a struc-tural allograft is recommended if a wedge is removed.

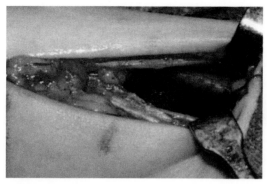

Fig. 1. Distal tibia bone graft harvest.

REAMER-IRRIGATOR-ASPIRATOR

A reamer-irrigator-aspirator (RIA) is used to obtain autologous cancellous graft and is a new technique. This graft can be used with a tibiotalocalcaneal arthrodesis as the intramedullary nail canal is created. A smaller amount can also be obtained through reaming of the fibula. It is important to make sure that the reamer diameter is appropriate for the diameter of the intramedullary canal. Nodzo and colleagues[27] evaluated iliac crest bone graft with RIA. They found that RIA showed significantly lower nonunion rates, and no patient undergoing RIA had chronic pain at the harvest site compared with 2 with the iliac crest bone graft.

BONE MARROW ASPIRATE

Bone marrow aspirate is used to promote bone repair by delivering pluripotent mesenchymal cells to the surgical site to have them differentiate into osteoblasts. Bone marrow aspirate is less invasive than harvesting autologous bone graft. The harvest is less invasive than iliac crest bone graft (ICBG) harvest, and it can be collected under local anesthetic. Bone marrow aspirate can be obtained from the proximal tibia around the Gerdy tubercle, distal tibia, or the calcaneus. There is a wide variety of live cells, including endothelial progenitor cells, mesenchymal stem cells, hematopoietic stem cells, and other progenitor cells, as well as growth factors, including platelet-derived growth factor, bone morphogenetic protein, transforming growth factor-B, vascular endothelial growth factor, interleukin (IL)-8, and IL-1

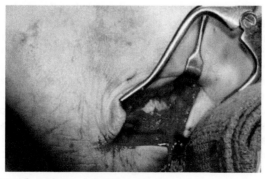

Fig. 2. Lateral incision for calcaneal graft harvest site.

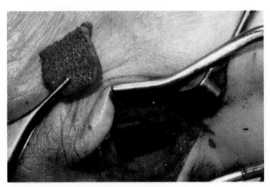

Fig. 3. Calcaneal corticocancellous autologous graft.

receptor antagonist.[7,28–31] Hyer and colleagues[32] found that some harvest locations have higher concentrations than others. Aspirate obtained from the anterior iliac crest had much higher concentrations of osteoblastic progenitor cells compared with the tibia or calcaneus.

Harvesting of bone marrow aspirate has a low complication rate. Roukis and colleagues[33] performed a multicenter, retrospective, observational cohort study of 530 subjects. All subjects underwent harvest of bone marrow aspiration from various sites in the lower extremity. All procedures were determined to be successful, with no infection, nerve injury, wound healing, or iatrogenic fractures.[34,35]

ALLOGRAFT

Demineralized bone matrix (DBM) is a type of allograft that has been processed to remove the mineralization but retains growth factors and proteins. The importance of DBM containing its original growth factors is to incorporate the undifferentiated cells into the osteoblasts and promote bone healing.[36]

It has been shown that antibiotics and freeze drying are both safe options that do not diminish the effects of the graft.[37,38] However, some sterilization techniques using gamma radiation, formaldehyde, or ethylene oxide can negate the osteoinductive properties of the DBM. There is no US Food and Drug Administration–regulated sterilization process for DBM, which causes an array of products with very little standardization.[36,39]

Because of the variation in the sterilization process, standardization of DBM is difficult and lacking, which is something that surgeons need to be aware of. DBM can be prepared many different ways, and has been shown to be effective in previous studies. However, only a few of these studies are specific to foot and ankle surgery.[40]

One study evaluated the effectiveness of DBM versus ICBGs in subtalar fusions and triple arthrodesis cases. Seven out of 8 patients with DBM in subtalar fusions achieved satisfactory healing and 1 had a nonunion radiographically but achieved pain relief. Three out of 3 patients obtained union with ICBG. For the triple arthrodesis group, 13 out of 15 healed with ICBGs and 29 out of 29 healed with DBM. Between the groups, time to achieve union was similar (3–4 months). The DBM group had reduced blood loss because the need for an autograft was eliminated. This study concluded DBM functioned as well as ICBGs and decreased donor site morbidity, blood loss, cost, and postoperative pain.[40] The investigators did mention that factors not affected by DBM included operating time and length of stay, but they believe these might be attributed to the study being conducted in an academic center. DBM was recommended by these investigators, and they suggested that it may be useful in mid-foot fusion as well.

Another study examined DBM putty and DBM with crushed cancellous allograft in ankle/hindfoot fusion.[41] The DBM putty group had a nonunion in 5 out of 38 of the patients, whereas the DBM with crushed cancellous allograft group had a nonunion in 2 out of 26 of the patients. Both groups went on to have either posttraumatic arthritis or other disorders in the patients with nonunion, but the study concluded that there was no difference in the fusion rates between the 2 substances, and the nonunion rate they achieved was very similar to the overall nonunion rate for hindfoot fusions using ICBGs.

Crosby and colleagues[42] studied arthroscopic ankle fusion with a slurry composed of DBM and iliac crest bone marrow. This study showed a radiographic union rate of 74%, with a clinical fusion rate of 93% at 5.5 months (other studies measured union rates at 1 year). This cohort revealed a high complication rate of 55%, which is within the 28% to 60% complication rate determined by other literature. This study concluded that the addition of DBM to bone marrow was not effective in improving the fusion rate, and the investigators recommended against using a DBM slurry.

The Michelson and Curl[40] study was the only one that recommended the use of DBM for hindfoot fusions. The other studies referenced did not necessarily advise avoiding DBM for foot and ankle fusions, but they concluded that using DBM was not effective in improving fusion rates for hindfoot surgery. The literature on the use of DBM and foot surgery is still lacking, and more studies need to be conducted to try to get a standardization of this allograft.

Bone Graft Substitutes

When considering the use of bone graft substitutes, it is important to remember that these are osteoconductive but not osteoinductive.[43] The 2 types of bone graft substitutes that have been found to be the most beneficial are coralline hydroxyapatite and a combination of hydroxyapatite, tricalcium phosphate (TCP), ceramic acid, and fibrillar collagen.[37] The combination bone graft substitute is made up of 65% hydroxyapatite, 35% TCP, and ceramic beads made of fibrillar bovine collagen, and combined with autogenous bone marrow. A study involving 267 subjects compared the combination graft with ICBGs for long bone fractures.[38] The results did not show any difference in radiographs comparing the two in more than 90% of subjects. The combination graft was also found to shorten operating time, determining that it aids in cost-effectiveness. Overall, it was determined that this graft was a safe and effective alternative to ICBGs in acute long bone fractures.[38,43] However, future research needs to further investigate the long-term effects of these bone graft substitutes and specifically study the foot and ankle in more depth.[37] Bone graft substitutes have the same porous properties as bone and thus can substitute well in the place of bone in terms of strength of the grafts.[37] However, without having collagen to support the structure of the substitute, they do not compare with the strength of bone when the grafts are first inserted. Over time, the grafts do surpass the strength of bone once they have had time to integrate into the structure of the bone. Another study investigated 40 subjects, all of whom had had tibial plateau fractures.[44] It compared 20 subjects who had coralline hydroxyapatite inserted with 20 subjects who had autografts used. There was no significant difference found between these patients when comparing their radiographs or postoperation clinical assessments. It was concluded that coralline hydroxyapatite is a safe and effective bone void filling alternative to cancellous autograft. In an additional review article, coralline hydroxyapatite grafts were recommended as a good alternative option compared with autogenous bone graft based on their biocompatibility, biodegradability, and safety.[37] This review found no difference in complications with the grafts either. From this information, it can be concluded that bone graft substitutes are a viable option.[43] There is still a chance that bone graft substitutes can induce an immune response in the body because of the presence of a foreign substance. This reaction can cause inflammation, infections, and other hazardous effects. A newer review from 2017 concluded that studies involving the bone substitutes calcium sulfate and calcium phosphate for intra-articular calcaneal fractures have yielded good clinical results in maintaining articular reduction and fracture union, and have produced minimal complications.[45] This review concluded that the use of these bone graft substitutes is supported by fair evidence to treat intra-articular calcaneal fractures. With all this information known to date, more extensive studies on bone graft substitutes ae still needed, focusing on the foot and ankle specifically. There are many different bone graft substitute options available that need further research as well.

DISCLOSURE

S.T. Grambart is a partner BESPA Global. The authors have no conflicts of interest in relation to this article.

REFERENCES

1. Giannoudis PV, Einhorn TA, Marsh D. Fracture healing: the diamond concept. Injury 2007;38(Suppl 4):S3–6.
2. Bibbo C, Hatfield PS. Platelet-rich plasma concentrate to augment bone fusion. Foot Ankle Clin 2010;15(4):641–9.
3. Gandhi A, Bibbo C, Pinzur M, et al. The role of platelet-rich plasma in foot and ankle surgery. Foot Ankle Clin 2005;10(4):621–37, viii.
4. Roberts TT, Rosenbaum AJ. Bone grafts, bone substitutes and orthobiologics: the bridge between basic science and clinical advancements in fracture healing. Organogenesis 2012;8(4):114–24.
5. Calcei JG, Rodeo SA. Orthobiologics for bone healing. Clin Sports Med 2019; 38(1):79–95.
6. Haddad SL, Coetzee JC, Estok R, et al. Intermediate and long-term outcomes of total ankle arthroplasty and ankle arthrodesis. A systematic review of the literature. J Bone Joint Surg Am 2007;89(9):1899–905.
7. Easley ME, Trnka HJ, Schon LC, et al. Isolated subtalar arthrodesis. J Bone Joint Surg Am 2000;82(5):613–24.
8. Myers TG, Lowery NJ, Frykberg RG, et al. Ankle and hindfoot fusions: comparison of outcomes in patients with and without diabetes. Foot Ankle Int 2012; 33(1):20–8.
9. Khan SN, Cammisa FP Jr, Sandhu HS, et al. The biology of bone grafting. J Am Acad Orthop Surg 2005;13(1):77–86.
10. Myeroff C, Archdeacon M. Autogenous bone graft: donor sites and techniques. J Bone Joint Surg Am 2011;93(23):2227–36.
11. Finkemeier CG. Bone-grafting and bone-graft substitutes. J Bone Joint Surg Am 2002;84(3):454–64.
12. Gazdag AR, Lane JM, Glaser D, et al. Alternatives to autogenous bone graft: efficacy and indications. J Am Acad Orthop Surg 1995;3(1):1–8.
13. Sen MK, Miclau T. Autologous iliac crest bone graft: should it still be the gold standard for treating nonunions? Injury 2007;38(Suppl 1):S75–80.

14. Bauer TW, Muschler GF. Bone graft materials. An overview of the basic science. Clin Orthop Relat Res 2000;371:10–27.
15. Olsen BS, Vaesel MT, Sojbjcrg JO. Treatment of midshaft clavicular nonunion with plate fixation and autologous bone grafting. J Shoulder Elbow Surg 1995;4(5): 337–44.
16. Bradbury N, Hutchinson J, Hahn D, et al. Clavicular nonunion. 31/32 healed after plate fixation and bone grafting. Acta Orthop Scand 1996;67(4):367–70.
17. Sanders R. Displaced intra-articular fractures of the calcaneus. J Bone Joint Surg Am 2000;82(2):225–50.
18. Cypher TJ, Grossman JP. Biological principles of bone graft healing. J Foot Ankle Surg 1996;35(5):413–7.
19. Mendicino RW, Leonheart E, Shromoff P. Techniques for harvesting autogenous bone graft of the lower extremity. J Foot Ankle Surg 1996;35(5):428–35.
20. Kakar S, Shin AY. Vascularized bone grafting from the dorsal distal radius for Kienbock's disease: technique, indications and review of the literature. Chir Main 2010;29(Suppl 1):S104–11.
21. DeOrio JK, Farber DC. Morbidity associated with anterior iliac crest bone grafting in foot and ankle surgery. Foot Ankle Int 2005;26(2):147–51.
22. Arrington ED, Smith WJ, Chambers HG, et al. Complications of iliac crest bone graft harvesting. Clin Orthop Relat Res 1996;329:300–9.
23. Younger EM, Chapman MW. Morbidity at bone graft donor sites. J Orthop Trauma 1989;3(3):192–5.
24. Chiodo CP, Hahne J, Wilson MG, et al. Histological differences in iliac and tibial bone graft. Foot Ankle Int 2010;31(5):418–22.
25. Miller CP, Chiodo CP. Autologous bone graft in foot and ankle surgery. Foot Ankle Clin 2016;21(4):825–37.
26. Saltrick KR, Caron M, Grossman J. Utilization of autogenous corticocancellous bone graft from the distal tibia for reconstructive surgery of the foot and ankle. J Foot Ankle Surg 1996;35(5):406–12.
27. Nodzo SR, Kaplan NB, Hohman DW, et al. A radiographic and clinical comparison of reamer-irrigator-aspirator versus iliac crest bone graft in ankle arthrodesis. Int Orthop 2014;38(6):1199–203.
28. DiGiovanni CW, Lin SS, Baumhauer JF, et al. Recombinant human platelet-derived growth factor-BB and beta-tricalcium phosphate (rhPDGF-BB/beta-TCP): an alternative to autogenous bone graft. J Bone Joint Surg Am 2013; 95(13):1184–92.
29. Frey C, Halikus NM, Vu-Rose T, et al. A review of ankle arthrodesis: predisposing factors to nonunion. Foot Ankle Int 1994;15(11):581–4.
30. O'Connor KM, Johnson JE, McCormick JJ, et al. Clinical and operative factors related to successful revision arthrodesis in the foot and ankle. Foot Ankle Int 2016;37(8):809–15.
31. Cottom JM, Plemmons BS. Bone marrow aspirate concentrate and its uses in the foot and ankle. Clin Podiatr Med Surg 2018;35(1):19–26.
32. Hyer CF, Berlet GC, Bussewitz BW, et al. Quantitative assessment of the yield of osteoblastic connective tissue progenitors in bone marrow aspirate from the iliac crest, tibia, and calcaneus. J Bone Joint Surg Am 2013;95(14): 1312–6.
33. Roukis TS, Hyer CF, Philbin TM, et al. Complications associated with autogenous bone marrow aspirate harvest from the lower extremity: an observational cohort study. J Foot Ankle Surg 2009;48(6):668–71.

34. Schade VL, Roukis TS. Percutaneous bone marrow aspirate and bone graft harvesting techniques in the lower extremity. Clin Podiatr Med Surg 2008;25(4):733–42, x.

35. Schweinberger MH, Roukis TS. Percutaneous autologous bone marrow harvest from the calcaneus and proximal tibia: surgical technique. J Foot Ankle Surg 2007;46(5):411–4.

36. Boyce T, Edwards J, Scarborough N. Allograft bone. The influence of processing on safety and performance. Orthop Clin North Am 1999;30(4):571–81.

37. Elsinger EC, Leal L. Coralline hydroxyapatite bone graft substitutes. J Foot Ankle Surg 1996;35(5):396–9.

38. Cornell CN, Lane JM, Chapman M, et al. Multicenter trial of Collagraft as bone graft substitute. J Orthop Trauma 1991;5(1):1–8.

39. Ijiri S, Yamamuro T, Nakamura T, et al. Effect of sterilization on bone morphogenetic protein. J Orthop Res 1994;12(5):628–36.

40. Michelson JD, Curl LA. Use of demineralized bone matrix in hindfoot arthrodesis. Clin Orthop Relat Res 1996;325:203–8.

41. Thordarson DB, Kuehn S. Use of demineralized bone matrix in ankle/hindfoot fusion. Foot Ankle Int 2003;24(7):557–60.

42. Crosby LA, Yee TC, Formanek TS, et al. Complications following arthroscopic ankle arthrodesis. Foot Ankle Int 1996;17(6):340–2.

43. Arner JW, Santrock RD. A historical review of common bone graft materials in foot and ankle surgery. Foot Ankle Spec 2014;7(2):143–51.

44. Bucholz RW, Carlton A, Holmes RE. Hydroxyapatite and tricalcium phosphate bone graft substitutes. Orthop Clin North Am 1987;18(2):323–34.

45. Wee J, Thevendran G. The role of orthobiologics in foot and ankle surgery: allogenic bone grafts and bone graft substitutes. EFORT Open Rev 2017;2(6):272–80.

Biologics for Tendon Surgery

Erin Nelson, DPM[a],*, Nephi E.H. Jones, DPM, PGY2[b], Mary Brandt, BA[a]

KEYWORDS

- Tendon surgery • Tendon biologics • Amnion graft

KEY POINTS

- An understanding of the anatomy and three phases of tendon healing is important in tendon repair.
- Current products being utilized in tendon surgery include amnion grafts, dermal allografts, tendon allograft and platelet rich plasma.
- There is potential for further research with the application of new products with tendon surgery.

INTRODUCTION

Technology continues to evolve at a rapid rate, and biologics is an area of continued research and new product development. This article summarizes the available biologics through literature review that is currently recommended with a focus on tendon surgery. The article reviews the anatomy and physiology of tendon healing with the application of biologics of tendon surgery.

TENDON ANATOMY

A tendon is the anatomic structure that allows the forces created by muscle to be transferred to bone and establish movement. In order to do so, tendons require a great amount of tensile strength, which is attributable to the high amounts of type 1 collagen present in the extracellular matrix.[1] Docheva and colleagues[2] state that type 1 collagen is approximately 95% of the total collagen. Type 3 collagen is the second most common; however, it is the first type to be produced in excess when damage occurs to a tendon. The extracellular matrix also consists of a ground substance, elastin, and inorganic compounds. Tenocytes are cells that surround collagen fibers and are responsible for synthesizing the ground substance. It is made up of large amounts of water, hyaluronan, proteoglycans, and glycoproteins that work to structurally reinforce the collagen fibers. Tenocytes also synthesize procollagen and play a large role in the healing process.[1]

[a] Des Moines University, 3200 Grand Avenue, Des Moines, IA 50312, USA; [b] Unitypoint Health - Iowa Methodist Medical Center, 1200 Pleasant Street, Des Moines, IA 50309, USA
* Corresponding author.
E-mail address: Erin.nelson@dmu.edu

Clin Podiatr Med Surg 37 (2020) 601–608
https://doi.org/10.1016/j.cpm.2020.03.013
0891-8422/20/© 2020 Elsevier Inc. All rights reserved.

The structure of a tendon is formed in a hierarchal manner that begins with tropo-collagen molecules that cross-link to create fibrils. Fibrils are the smallest structural unit of a tendon, and they aggregate to form fibers.[2] Bundles of fibers are surrounded by endotendon to create fascicles. Endotendon is a loose connective tissue that contains blood vessels, nerves, and lymphatics that run throughout the course of the tendon. In the same way, fascicles are condensed together and surrounded by epitendon. Epitendon is continuous with the endotendon septa, also containing blood vessels, nerves, and lymphatics.[3] Tendons that act in a straight course have a paratenon that is present superficially around the endotendon. When present, the epitendon and paratenon form a 2-layered synovial sheath called the peritendon. However, many of the tendons in the foot and ankle contain true tendon sheaths that are needed to overcome the frictional forces caused by the curved path the tendons take.[1]

Blood supply to the tendons can be achieved in a variety of ways, primarily from tendon sheaths in the foot and ankle. This complex receives nutrients via diffusion from the blood vessels and synovium from the nearby muscle. Blood vessels that surround the tendon also continue to flow proximally at its osteotendinous junction and distally at the myotendinous junction. The paratenon can be a source of blood supply to tendons when present as well. The vasculature enters the paratenon at multiple locations to form a network of capillaries. The blood supply to tendons is a crucial part of the healing process, which can be delayed in the ankle because most tendons are surrounded by sheaths rather than paratenon.[1]

TENDON HEALING

Once a tendon's integrity is disrupted, the body's healing process starts. The healing process has been described as having both intrinsic and extrinsic models. The intrinsic model involves migration of inflammatory cells within the tendon itself when the damage occurs within the tendon. During the extrinsic portion, tenocytes are attracted to the site of injury from the periphery.[4] From there, the healing process is broken down into 3 phases. The phases are the inflammatory, the proliferative, and the remodeling or maturation. The inflammatory phase lasts up to 4 to 7 days. The formation of a hematoma begins as the ends of the tendon retract. Proinflammatory cytokines draw in cells such as neutrophils, platelets, and mast cells from extrinsic peritendinous tissue.[1] A vascular network begins to form, and fibroblasts start to fill in the tendon gap. Near the fifth day, the fibroblasts start to synthesize collagen, predominately type 3, and will continue to form over the next few weeks. In the following weeks, when collagen is synthesized, tenocytes become the predominant cell type.[4]

In the subsequent 7 to 14 days, the proliferative phase occurs. During this time, there is an increase in extracellular matrix (ECM) factors, specifically type 3 collagen.[2] The process is done in a sporadic manner, and although the gap in the tendon closes, the connection is not yet strong at this time. It is in the final maturation, or remodeling, phase whereby collagen fibers align and begin to cross-link.[1] Type 1 collagen gradually replaces type 3, but never returns to the amount that healthy tissue has. The remodeling is a slow process as the body begins to form an organized scar. In 6 months' time, the tissue components of the scar are very similar to healthy tissue, but the maturation phase continues for a year or more. Because the cellular components of the tendon never reach the levels that they once were, there is a lack of tensile strength that the body tries to compensate for. There can ultimately be stiffening of the tendon that diminishes the movement of the tendon.[2]

ALLOGRAFT

Human amniotic membranes have been used to manage burns, ulcers, tendon/nerve repair, and infected wounds since as early as the 1900s.[5–11] In 1950, Troensegaard-Hansen[12] published a 6-patient series on the successful application of amniotic membrane to treat chronic skin ulcers. The lack of complete understanding of the mechanism of repair opened the door to further investigations and more studies into the use of amniotic allograft. In recent decades, there has been an uptrend in the availability and uses of amnion and/or chorion grafts. A few examples of how these products are currently being used are for acute wounds often related to trauma or burns, for chronic ulceration, tendon, and nerve repair, and for the cornea.[11,13] Using amnion with wound healing has promoted a decrease in wound recurrence, improved healing time, and improved revascularization.[13,14]

The human placenta is composed of an amnion layer that interfaces with the fetus and a chorion layer that is the outer layer and has maternal contact.[13] There is a spongy layer between the amnion layer and chorion layer that contains collagen, proteoglycans, and glycoproteins.[13] The amniotic layer is an avascular structure that functions to help regulate metabolic activities and also has collagen types I, III, V, and VI.[13] It can promote anti-inflammatory properties through suppression of interleukin-1α, interleukin-1β, and matrix metalloproteases. The amnion and chorion layers both contain growth factors, including insulin-like growth factor, transforming growth factor-beta (TGF-β), fibroblast growth factor, vascular endothelial growth factor (VEGF), and platelet-derived growth factor (PDGF). These growth factors aid in activating cellular proliferation, differentiation, and cell migration,[15,16] which can ultimately assist in tendon repair.

The chorion layer, which is also avascular, is 4 times the thickness of the amniotic membrane. The chorion layer also helps to regulate metabolic activity through similar growth factors as the amnion layer. It also contains collagen types I, III, IV, V, and VI.[13] Through this, the combination of the amnion and chorion layers can contain 5 times the growth factors of the single amnion layer.[16] Because of their avascularity, the layers are able to possess the anti-inflammatory and antimicrobial properties and are low immunogenicity. New advances in the ability of freezing and preserving sections of the membrane have led to further expansion in its clinical use.

A method of dehydration and sterilization of the amniotic membranes is called PURION and can be performed after extensive screening of donors. This process separates, cleans, and reassembles the layers and then dehydrates them to maintain the healing components. This product then must be stored in a frozen state.[13,17]

Placental-derived allografts traditionally have been used in sheets, but an alternate approach for use in tendon repair is to use an amniotic suspension graft (ASA) made up of amniotic membrane and amniotic fluid cells.[15] Kimmerling and colleagues[15] determined that ASA resulted in increased cell density, more robust cell migration, matrix deposition, and reduced inflammation.

Indications of using the grafts for tendons are still in investigational stages. Tendon grafts can be applied as an onlay graft (graft laid upon or wrapped around the tendon and sutured in place), inlay graft (a strip of graft material is placed within the substance of the tendon parallel to the tendon fibers), or any of a variety of weaving techniques, according to Branch (**Fig. 1**).[18]

As previously stated, human amniotic membranes have been used to manage burns, ulcers, and infected wounds, and there is limited published research on the use

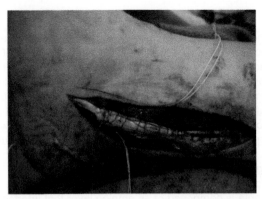

Fig. 1. Peroneal longus allograft for reconstruction of a peroneal brevis and longus rupture.

in tendon injuries and repair. With that being said, the growth factors and ECM found in amniotic membrane show great promise in assisting in tendon repair and healing (**Fig. 2**).

GraftJacket

GraftJacket (Wright Medical, Memphis, TN) is a human dermal allograft matrix used primarily to provide supplemental support, protection, and reinforcement of tendon and ligament tissue. GraftJacket is a dermal collagen matrix that readily incorporates into the surgical repair. The material is acellular and has the ability to be freeze-dried; this increases its clinical use. Like many other matrices and allografts, it acts as a scaffold for host cell growth, migration, and revascularization.

Barber and colleagues[19] performed a cadaveric study comparing primary repair of acute Achilles tendon rupture with primary repair with human dermal allograft

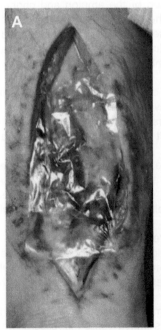
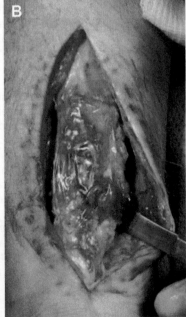

Fig. 2. (*A, B*) Achilles tendon with amniotic membrane.

augmentation (GraftJacket) to determine if there would be a significant difference in increased strength and stiffness of the repair. They reported the ultimate failure load in the control group was 217 ± 31 N compared with 455 ± 76.5 N in the GraftJacket group (P<.001). The mean stiffness in the control group was 4.3 ± 0.83 N/mm, which was significantly less than the 12.99 ± 5.34 N/mm in the GraftJacket group (P = .002). They concluded there was significantly increased repair strength and stiffness with GraftJacket augmentation. They hypothesize that this could lead to more aggressive and early rehabilitation and return to full activities.

Baumhauer and O'Brien[20] published a review on the considerations for lateral ankle instability and discussed augmenting the modified Bröstrom-Gould technique to reinforce the repair to help reduce inversion, the likelihood of reinjury, and correcting the subtalar joint component of the instability. Baumhauer and O'Brien recommend incorporating a dermal allograft into the surgical repair of lateral ankle ligament and tendon repairs to assist in providing increased strength, stiffness, and cellular migration into the repair.

PLATELET-RICH PLASMA

When a tendon sustains an injury, a variety of growth factors are activated in stimulating healing, which leads to increased cellularity and tissue volume. During the early phases of healing, there is understandably an increase in expression of important growth factors. Literature review shows basic fibroblast growth factor (bFGF), bone morphogenetic protein (BMP)-12, -13, -14, connective tissue growth factor, insulin-like growth factor (IGF)-1, PDGF, TGF-β, and VEGF are most important in tendon healing.[21–24] Platelet-rich plasma (PRP) contains these important tendon-healing growth factors and is already in clinical use for tendon injuries and repair.[25–29] The literature surrounding the efficacy of the use of PRP in tendon repair and injury is somewhat contradictory, with some studies reporting successful use and others reporting no change or failure of its use.

Gosens and colleagues[29] reported significant pain reduction in 36 patients with patellar tendinopathy after PRP injection.

de Almeida and colleagues[30] conducted a prospective randomized controlled study of 27 patients who underwent anterior cruciate ligament (ACL) reconstruction with PRP injection of the patellar tendon graft, resulting in reduced pain and smaller defect size in MRI controls after 6 months.

Seijas and colleagues[31] compared PRP with no PRP use during ACL reconstruction with patellar tendon graft and reported faster remodeling of the patellar tendon graft after use of PRP.

Aspenberg and Virchenko[25] conducted a study using rats whereby a 3-mm section of Achilles tendon was resected with percutaneous administration of PRP 6 hours after transection. They reported increased tendon callus and strength by approximately 30% after 1 week, which continued for up to 3 weeks after injection.

In comparison, Schepull and colleagues[32] conducted a randomized single-blind study using PRP after acute Achilles tendon rupture repair in patients. They concluded there was no improvement in healing in human Achilles tendon repair with the use of PRP.

de Vos and colleagues[33] conducted a randomized control trial on the use of PRP in chronic Achilles tendinopathy and reported no differences in pain or activity level between patients treated with PRP or saline. In addition, de Vos and colleagues[34] conducted a systematic review on treating lateral epicondylar tendinopathy using PRP injections and again found no evidence of efficacy using PRP. Hall and colleagues[35] conducted a similar review and concluded that PRP should be reserved for refractory

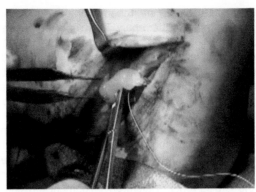

Fig. 3. Platelet-rich plasma (PRP) clot used for revision repair of a peroneal tendon repair.

cases of lateral epicondylar tendinopathy, but not for other tendinopathies or tendon repair.

With the lack of agreement on the use of PRP in tendinopathy, tendon injuries, or tendon repair surgeries, it is difficult to draw strong conclusions on its efficacy or when it should be used (**Fig. 3**).

RESTRATA

A new available option is a synthetic resorbable nanofiber wound matrix (Restrata; Acera Surgical, St Louis, MO, USA). The matrix is an electrospun fully resorbable nanofiber scaffold composed of 2 synthetic polymers: polyglactin 910 poly(lactic-co-glycolic acid) (10:90) and polydioxanone. These materials are biocompatible and commonly found in existing medical products (eg, resorbable sutures).[36] The matrix allows for cellular migration, oxygen permeation, and exudate management. Resorption rates of the product are tailored to match the rate of new tissue formation, which dissolves via hydrolysis within approximately 30 to 45 days.[36] Although it does not contain growth factors like allografts, it does offer ECM to allow for cellular migration and structure for tendon healing. The goal of tendon repair is to restore strength and function of the tendon while eliminating adhesions and scarring during the healing process. This product is designed to assist in normal cellular migration (tenocytes in tendon repair) and help reduce fibrotic ingrowth leading to reduced adhesions. More research is being undertaken to determine the efficacy and viability of this product.

DISCLOSURE

The authors have nothing to disclose.

REFERENCES

1. Platt M. Tendon repair and healing. Clin Podiatric Med Surg 2005;22(4):553–60.

2. Docheva D, Mueller SA, Majewski M, et al. Biologics for tendon repair. Adv Drug Deliv Rev 2015;84:222–39.

3. Riley G. The pathogenesis of tendinopathy. A molecular perspective. Rheumatology 2003;43(2):131–42.

4. Maffulli N, Moller H. Optimization of tendon healing. In: Maffulli N, Renström P, Leadbetter WB, editors. Tendon injuries: Basic Science and Clinical Medicine. London: Springer; 2005. p. 304–6.

5. Mowry K, Bonvallet P, Bellis S. Enhanced skin regeneration using a novel amniotic-derived tissue graft. Wounds 2017;29(9):277–85.

6. Gruss JS, Jirsch DW. Human amniotic membrane: a versatile wound dressing. Can Med Assoc J 1978;118(10):1237–46.

7. Mermet I, Pottier N, Sainthillier JM, et al. Use of amniotic membrane transplantation in the treatment of venous leg ulcers. Wound Repair Regen 2007;15(4): 459–64.

8. Sawhney CP. Amniotic membrane as a biological dressing in the management of burns. Burns 1989;15(5):339–42.

9. Davis J. Skin transplantation with a review of 550 cases at the Johns Hopkins Hospital. Johns Hopkins Med J 1910;15:307–96.

10. Stern M. The grafting of preserved amniotic membrane to burned and ulcerated surfaces, substituting skin grafts. JAMA 1913;60(13):973–4.

11. Fairbairn NG, Randolph MA, Redmond RW. The clinical applications of human amnion in plastic surgery. J Plast Reconstr Aesthet Surg 2014;67(5):662–75.

12. Troensegaard-Hansen E. Amniotic grafts in chronic skin ulceration. Lancet 1950; 255(6610):859–60.

13. Lei J, Priddy LB, Lim JJ, et al. Dehydrated human amnion/chorion membrane (dHACM) allografts as a therapy for orthopedic tissue repair. Tech Orthopedics 2017;32(3):149–57.

14. Brigido SA. Emerging insights on using acellular amniotic scaffolds to treat periarticular tendon tears. Podiatry Today 2016;29(7):26–30.

15. Kimmerling K, McQuilling J, Staples M, et al. Tenocyte cell density, migration, and extracellular matrix deposition with amniotic suspension allograft. J Orthop Res 2018;37(2):412–20.

16. Przybylski M. Amniotic membrane allografts in the outpatient wound clinic: current practice guidelines & modalities. Wound Clin 2018;12(7):10–2.

17. Purion process. Available at: https://mimedx.com/purion-process/. Accessed April 14, 2020.

18. Branch JP. A tendon graft weave using acellular dermal matrix for repair of the Achilles tendon and other foot and ankle tendons. J Foot Ankle Surg 2011;(50): 257–65.

19. Barber FA, McGarry JE, Herbert MA, et al. A biomechanical study of Achilles tendon repair augmentation using GraftJacket matrix. Foot Ankle Int 2008; 29(3):329–33.

20. Baumhauer JF, O'Brien T. Surgical considerations in the treatment of ankle instability. J Athl Train 2002;37(4):458–62.

21. Wurgler-Hauri CC, Dourte LM, Baradet TC, et al. Soslowsky temporal expression of 8 growth factors in tendon-to-bone healing in a rat supraspinatus model. J Shoulder Elbow Surg 2007;16:S198–203.

22. Chen CH, Cao Y, Wu YF, et al. Tendon healing in vivo: gene expression and production of multiple growth factors in early tendon healing period. J Hand Surg Am 2008;33:1834–42.

23. Kobayashi M, Itoi E, Minagawa H, et al. Expression of growth factors in the early phase of supraspinatus tendon healing in rabbits. J Shoulder Elbow Surg 2006; 15:371–7.

24. Molloy T, Wang Y, Murrell G. The roles of growth factors in tendon and ligament healing. Sports Med 2003;33:381–94.

25. Aspenberg P, Virchenko O. Platelet concentrate injection improves Achilles tendon repair in rats. Acta Orthop Scand 2004;75:93–9.
26. Bosch G, van Schie HT, de Groot MW, et al. Effects of platelet-rich plasma on the quality of repair of mechanically induced core lesions in equine superficial digital flexor tendons: a placebo-controlled experimental study. J Orthop Res 2010;28: 211–7.
27. Majewski M, Ochsner PE, Liu F, et al. Accelerated healing of the rat Achilles tendon in response to autologous conditioned serum. Am J Sports Med 2009; 37:2117–25.
28. Schnabel LV, Mohammed HO, Miller BJ, et al. Platelet rich plasma (PRP) enhances anabolic gene expression patterns in flexor digitorum superficialis tendons. J Orthop Res 2007;25:230–40.
29. Gosens T, Den Oudsten BL, Fievez E, et al. Pain and activity levels before and after platelet-rich plasma injection treatment of patellar tendinopathy: a prospective cohort study and the influence of previous treatments. Int Orthop 2012;36: 1941–6.
30. de Almeida AM, Demange MK, Sobrado MF, et al. Patellar tendon healing with platelet-rich plasma: a prospective randomized controlled trial. Am J Sports Med 2012;40:1282–8.
31. Seijas R, Ares O, Catala J, et al. Magnetic resonance imaging evaluation of patellar tendon graft remodelling after anterior cruciate ligament reconstruction with or without platelet-rich plasma. J Orthop Surg (Hong Kong) 2013;21:10–4.
32. Schepull T, Kvist J, Norrman H, et al. Autologous platelets have no effect on the healing of human Achilles tendon ruptures: a randomized single-blind study. Am J Sports Med 2011;39:38–47.
33. de Vos RJ, Weir A, van Schie HT, et al. Platelet-rich plasma injection for chronic Achilles tendinopathy: a randomized controlled trial. JAMA 2010;303:144–9.
34. de Vos RJ, Windt J, Weir A. Strong evidence against platelet-rich plasma injections for chronic lateral epicondylar tendinopathy: a systematic review. Br J Sports Med 2014;48:952–6.
35. Hall MP, Ward JP, Cardone DA. Platelet rich placebo? Evidence for platelet rich plasma in the treatment of tendinopathy and augmentation of tendon repair. Bull Hosp Jt Dis 2013;71:54–9.
36. MacEwan MR, MacEan S, Wright AP, et al. Efficacy of a nanofabricated electrospun wound matrix in treating full-thickness cutaneous wounds in a porcine model. Wounds 2018;30(2):E21–4.

Moving?

Make sure your subscription moves with you!

To notify us of your new address, find your **Clinics Account Number** (located on your mailing label above your name), and contact customer service at:

Email: journalscustomerservice-usa@elsevier.com

800-654-2452 (subscribers in the U.S. & Canada)
314-447-8871 (subscribers outside of the U.S. & Canada)

Fax number: 314-447-8029

Elsevier Health Sciences Division
Subscription Customer Service
3251 Riverport Lane
Maryland Heights, MO 63043

*To ensure uninterrupted delivery of your subscription, please notify us at least 4 weeks in advance of move.

Printed and bound by CPI Group (UK) Ltd, Croydon, CR0 4YY

03/10/2024

01040481-0019